BEAU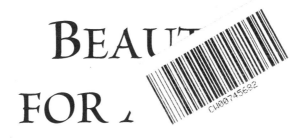
FOR

Letters from a Mother's Heart

To Eric & Monika, my sweet
brother & sister in law.
Isaiah 61 v 3.

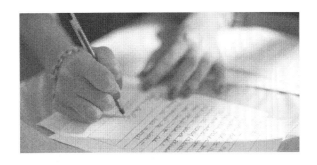

LAURA JOHN

Strategic Book Publishing and Rights Co.

Strategic Book Publishing and Rights Co.
12620 FM 1960, Suite A4-507
Houston, TX 77065
www.sbpra.com

ISBN: 978-1-62516-408-7

Cover design by Laura-Louisa Betts

Typography and page composition by J. K. Eckert & Company

This book is dedicated to my mother,

an amazing woman who has lived an extraordinary,

adventurous, God-filled life,

and my late father,

who was a man of exceptional talents,

perseverance, and faith.

The older I get, the more I forgive and understand.

Contents

Preface

Motherhood has been a rocky road for me, full of highs and lows. This book of letters reveals my feelings for my children and the events in our lives. In some cases, it has only been in hindsight that I could write these letters as in them I explore my emotions, my actions, and their consequences. They are from my heart.

Many times I have felt that my life and my relationships were but ashes. God's grace has replaced this with beauty. I still struggle with feelings of inadequacy as a parent, but there is no question that I love my children unconditionally.

In recent times, I have been able to talk to my older children about a few of the very painful experiences in their lives. In some cases our perceptions are very different. One of the differences is the concept of time. To a child, a week is an eternity; to a parent, it is but a blink of the eye. A child only understands their reality, but a parent is often aware of consequences and implications for the whole family. Like they say, there are two sides to every coin and relationships are far more complicated than coins!

I know my own parents' and sister's recollections of the circumstances surrounding my teenage pregnancy and subsequent abortion are at variance to mine. In the same way, my own children will perceive some of the events I talk about very differently from me. They have all had the opportunity to read the letters and have supported me in the writing of this book although at times they have found my account of the events to be very confronting. The theme of this book is one of redemption. I hope it shows that miracles still happen, gives encouragement to those readers who need it, and provides insight for others. For the sake of privacy, all the names in the book have been changed.

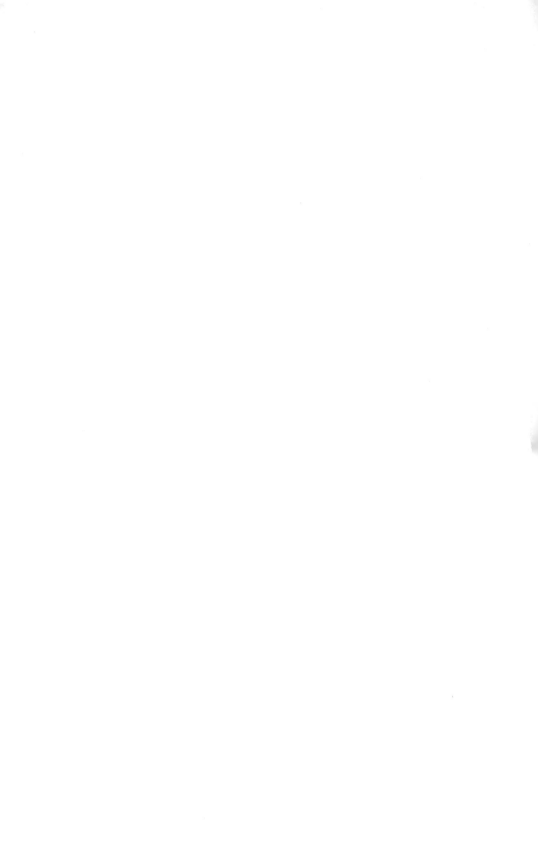

Acknowledgments

I thank my husband, Leroy, for his unfailing support of me in this venture. When I told him I wanted to write, he said, "Write." When I told him I needed my own laptop, he bought me one. When I needed time on my own, he held the fort at home. At all levels, he has given me encouragement in my writing. It is amazing that someone believes in my abilities the way he does.

It is even more amazing because he knows that in writing these letters I would be bound to expose some of our failures as parents, his and mine, and would go over some very painful ground from our past. I would highlight some of our imperfections, doubts, and inadequacies. In some cases, I never put into words the feelings I express in these letters. I hope he is pleased with the result. He is a very brave man and I love him dearly with all my heart.

Also, I would like to thank Laura-Louisa Betts, who was my unexpected and talented houseguest at the time this book was ready to be published, for working so closely with me to design and beautifully illustrate the front cover.

Finally, as Leroy would say, "Praise the Lord."

Chronology

1976	First unborn	Year of conception
1986	Daniel	Birth year
1987	Sally	Birth year
1997	Leo, stepson	Came into my life
1998	Lilly	Birth year
2000	Second unborn	Year of conception
2001	Third unborn	Year of conception
2003	Callum	Birth year

1

To the Child Who Started It All

Despair

Dear child,

The day your life ended started in Nairobi, Kenya and finished just outside London, England. I was seventeen years old when you were conceived. I was alone; I felt trapped. I was petrified, and I had no idea where to go and no one to turn to if I kept you. I aborted you in a blur. I loved you. I wanted you and I named you.

It has taken me a long time to write this letter although most of it has been in my head for a long, long time.

If you could speak to me, I expect that your first question would probably be "Why? Why did you get rid of me? Why didn't you want me? Why did you reject me even before I was born?"

So here goes; I did want you, but I felt I had no other option.

You were conceived in England where I studied for nearly two years. I lived with an auntie, uncle, and four cousins in a small three-bed council semi on a housing estate in Manchester. Your father was my first ever boyfriend. I thought I knew everything, but I knew very little about life, about people, about consequences and I most certainly knew nothing about sex. I thought I had all the answers, but you left me with only questions.

I was born in Congo, central Africa, and lived in Congo, England, Zambia, South Africa, and Kenya before I finally arrived in England age sixteen years and two months. I discovered I was pregnant whilst visiting my parents who were still living and working in Nairobi, Kenya.

It was an unplanned visit that came about because my mother fell off a kitchen cabinet whilst attempting to take down curtains for cleaning. She fell onto a concrete floor and had a neck injury that made her very dizzy. My father was very busy with his missionary work. At the time, he worked with displaced and refugee youth in Nairobi and could not care for her. My only surviving sister had just moved to Canada and was starting Bible College.

On the other hand, I just completed my "A" levels in England and was waiting for the results before getting a placement in an English teacher training college. I got on the plane with much trepidation, not the normal excitement I had before travel. I had not seen my parents for two years and would normally be excited by the reunion, but this time it was different.

My boyfriend did not want me to go and asked me to marry him before I left Manchester. I agreed, but in my heart I did not want to marry him.

Although we had only been going out for a few months, he had already shown me that he was violent, jealous, and manipulative. On one occasion, I tried to break off the relationship and he leaned over the banister on the second floor of the shopping center we were in and threatened to commit suicide if I ever left him.

When we first started dating, he completely bowled me over with his attention. I could not believe it when he asked me out. I was on cloud nine. My feet scarcely touched the ground. Several of the girls in my church youth group fancied him and he picked me. I was amazed and excited. He was very good-looking, older than me (twenty-two) and had long dark hair (very fashionable in 1976, believe it or not!) His name was Colin and every time I was with him, I felt excited and tingly. His mere touch gave me goose bumps. When we were apart, I ached to be with him and I thought about him 100 percent of the time. Surely this is love, I thought.

Several people started to warn me about him. Firstly, his older brother cautioned me to be very careful with him. He basically said that his brother was bad news and I should be very wary and not spend any time alone with him, that he was too old for me, and that he would try to get me into bed. Of course, I totally ignored this and other warnings.

At the time, the church I was attending joined with other churches in the United Kingdom for an annual conference at a Butlins holiday camp. I had been the year previously and had really enjoyed the holiday. (Not so much for the spiritual input as for the social side.) Most of the churches brought groups of young people with them and it became a chance for fun and romance with the opportunity to meet other young people from similar backgrounds from all around the United Kingdom and make new friends.

Colin and I both booked to go on the holiday. I booked into a chalet with some of the other girls and he booked into a chalet with three of his brothers. The week was great and I loved every minute. We spent nearly all our time together, only separating for sleep. A couple of times our kissing went a little farther than I really wanted, but I felt that I could handle the situation. Although Colin at this time said he was a Christian, he didn't really live the way I had been brought up to think that Christians lived. He smoked, drank alcohol, and swore. We never really spoke about anything religious. The camp was alcohol free for the week of the conference, as this was one of the requests of the church organization that booked the whole of the campus for the week, so I did not really get to see the true Colin at this time.

We returned to Manchester on a Saturday afternoon at the end of the week. The coach we were travelling on dropped us all at the church and from there, we made our separate ways home, arranging to meet up again later at the church before going on to a friend's house. Colin and I arranged to meet up a couple of hours later in Stockport town center, which was about halfway between our houses.

I expect you are wondering why I am telling you this. Well, it is to explain what happened next, which is really where you come in or at least the possibility of you comes in. Remember I said that at that time I knew nothing about sex; well I really did not know anything at all. Colin was my first boyfriend and the first boy I had ever kissed (excluding of course, some quick pecks under the mistletoe at Christmas or when the clock struck twelve on New Years Eve). Everyone I knew had "been out" with someone or was "going out" with someone. All of the four cousins I was living with were dating someone. I felt very left out.

My early teens were full of unrequited love. Most of the boys that I fancied only ever spoke to me to get an introduction to my sister, who was very popular with the boys. She was fully equipped sexually at ten years old with basically the same body shape that she has continued to have in her adult life. She has always had good looks of the Princess Diana variety with whom she has often been compared. I, on the other hand, did not get my periods until I was fourteen and was also as flat as a pancake up top until then. Once my periods did start, I lost them at age fifteen through very irregular eating patterns at boarding school in Kenya and had to be put on the pill temporarily to kick them back into action at sixteen. I felt fat and ugly and used to starve myself during the week at school and then eat only when I visited my parents every other weekend on a Saturday. I had worn glasses since the age of four and they were the bane of my life. Other kids at school used to ask me if I was blind because they were so thick they looked like the bottom of coke bottles.

Then along came contact lenses. What a transformation! I felt like a human being and I could actually see what my face looked like without glasses. Looking back at photographs of myself at that time, I now realize that I was neither fat nor ugly, just living in the shadow of my sister who was not only beautiful, but also seemed to be good at everything. Of course, the shadow was mostly of my own making.

Back to what happened next. I met Colin as arranged, but instead of continuing on to meet up with the rest of the young people at someone's house, Colin took me to a pub. I had never been inside a pub before so was quite intrigued. I felt a little nervous because I was not expecting this turn of events. I was definitely on unfamiliar territory and definitely not in control of the situation, but after all, I was nearly eighteen and eighteen is grown up, isn't it? I should be allowed to make my own decisions and this was quite exciting. I don't remember much about this part of the evening except that Colin bought me a few drinks that tasted rather strange, kind of sweet with a bit of a kick in them. He called them brandy and babychams. The only alcoholic drinks I had ever really heard of were beer and wine, so I figured this one must be okay because it was neither.

I knew about wine because the Bible talks about wine, only my parents had told me that there were two types of wine, alcoholic and non-alcoholic. They had told me that drinking the alcoholic wine was a sin. I had in fact tasted some alcoholic wine when I was sixteen, much to my mother's chagrin. It was on an occasion nearly two years earlier when I came to England to continue my education. My mother had accompanied me on the flight and we stayed with my grandparents for a couple of weeks until she left and went back to Kenya. During those weeks, we visited some of her family and it was whilst visiting with her older brother, Jock, and his wife, Jane, that I had tasted the wine. They had a bottle of wine on the table and had offered me some. When I accepted, my mother nearly choked on her food, but by that time my uncle had already poured it out, I tasted some. It didn't taste that bad and I wondered what all the fuss was about, but my mother forbade me to finish the glass. I expect my mother and her brother had a right old row after that as he would have known full well her views on alcohol and probably only offered me the wine to provoke her. My mother had signed the pledge (never to drink alcohol) when she was twelve, and later as a Christian missionary, she had agreed again never to drink alcohol. Her brother may have been aware of this, but obviously did not think about it at the time.

Enough about the wine incident. I guess I am including it here because it will give you an idea of my naivety and innocence. I didn't actually realize that I was drinking alcohol and I certainly didn't realize that I was drinking a strong alcoholic drink, much stronger than beer or wine. I remember Colin saying that he would get me a double brandy in the babycham because the drinks were quite little and doubles were better. I took his word for it because I was no longer feeling worried about not having stuck to the plan. I didn't care that we had not met our friends. When Colin suggested that we go back to where I was living and have some time alone whilst everyone else was still out, I was very happy to do so.

When we got in to the house, he started kissing me almost straight away. The next thing I knew, he was on top of me. He was pinning both my hands to the floor and his whole body was on top of me. I could not move. His mouth was over mine and I was trying to speak and tell him to stop, but couldn't get the words out. I felt really scared, but it was over in a few seconds. He jumped up and did his trousers up and told me to fix my clothes. I felt really confused. What had just happened? Had I had sex; was that it?

I asked him, "Why didn't you stop? I told you I didn't want to have sex."

He told me not to worry about it, and that we hadn't had sex; it was just a bit of fun. I stood up and rearranged my clothes. Everything seemed to have changed; he seemed a little distant even. I asked him again what had just happened, and he just told me that of course, we hadn't had sex.

Honestly, my dear child, at that point, I did not know that I had just had sex, nor did I realize that I had in fact been raped because it was non-consensual. It is only now, looking back, that I realize that my first real sexual experience was date rape and that plain old alcohol was used to loosen my inhibitions.

Over the next couple of months, more of these date rapes occurred. Once, when I had finally realized that these encounters were in fact sex, I strongly resisted. Because I did not wish to continue, he grabbed a kitchen knife and held it to my throat, saying it was my fault because I should not have turned him on. He also started accusing me of having sex with other people and saying that he didn't believe I had been a virgin because I had led him on. He said I really wanted to have sex even though I told him I didn't. He made me feel guilty for him forcing me to have sex.

On one occasion, he actually finished with me. I remember this clearly; we were standing under a street lamp not far from where I lived. He told me he did not want to go out with me anymore and that I was now free to go out with someone else at church. He then asked me whom I fancied and whom I planned to date once we were finished. He kept saying it was all right to tell him as he had now finished with me. He started naming guys from church one by one and saying that he thought I was after them because he had seen me looking at them or speaking to them or laughing at one of their jokes.

I told him I didn't have plans to go out with anyone else and that I was not involved with anyone else. After a while of intense questioning, he told me that he had only been testing me and that he had not finished with me. I was his; he was just trying to find out if I was lying to him or going behind his back with another guy. So my moment of freedom had passed, although it was probably never a moment of freedom, just a manipulation. Of course, I now realize how controlling that situation was and even at the time, I found it vaguely frightening and threatening. Why did he think that I was interested in anyone else? It was really puzzling, but I was beginning to realize that my relationship with him was not quite right, not healthy; it seemed to be based on mistrust. This relationship business was a lot more complicated than I realized at first. I don't know if it is like this with everyone, but I took my situation at that time as being normal. I had never had a boyfriend so maybe this was what it was like to have one; maybe you just didn't say what you felt, take each other at their word, and accept "yes" and "no" at their face value. Maybe it was just some kind of complicated game that I didn't know how to play and no one had given me the rules. Maybe there weren't any rules even!

I believed with all my heart that sex should only be between two people who were married. I also thought that sex would be beautiful and wonderful and this was neither of these. Often I would read my Bible, start to cry, pray, ask God to forgive me, and promise that I would not let it happen again. Of course, Colin had asked me to marry him before the first incident, but that didn't really count as the real deal. I struggled with my feelings. He scared me, but he told me he loved me and that he couldn't live without me. I tried to end the relationship, but he begged me to continue, threatening suicide.

I did not know whom to talk to; I gave up protesting, as it did not make any difference. I felt trapped. All this was happening whilst I was sitting for my "A" Level exams. I was in a total whirl and did very little revision. On the surface, everything was fine, but underneath, I was totally messed up. Colin and I continued to attend church, not just once a week, but every night of the week. I continued to go out with him, which seems strange to me looking back. I so desperately wanted to belong to someone, having felt abandoned most of my life and he was so intense.

I now recognize him as a sexual predator who groomed me and manipulated me. Sexual predators get the victim to think that what is going on is normal and okay at the same time making it a special secret even when the victim does not want to participate. This is what happened to me. Just as I did not know how to conduct myself in a relationship, I also did not know how to end the relationship, especially when we attended the same church and I would either have to leave or have to see him six nights a week. My auntie and uncle were great people, but they had no idea what was going on and neither did any of my cousins. I did not ever talk to any of them about what was going on or how I was feeling. I am sure they just assumed that everything was okay. I remember that my auntie had a talk with me one day and said that she and my uncle were a bit worried about your dad; they didn't feel that he was a good influence and they didn't want me to bring him to the house. This is probably the time I should have confided in her, but I felt threatened and backed off.

Life has curious twists and turns.

Out of the blue, a call came from my parents in Kenya. I was needed to go and look after my mother for a few months. They arranged the flights and it was indeed a way out of the situation, the only trouble was, my period was late.

When I arrived in Nairobi, I was confused and in emotional turmoil. It had been two years since I had left Kenya at just sixteen years of age. I really had no friends there any more as most of them had left Kenya at the same time as me, after graduation. My sister and I had attended an American-run school in the Rift Valley. Most of the students were the children of missionaries from all over East Africa; some even came from Congo and a few from South Africa. Only I and one other girl had gone to England and most of the rest had gone on to further education in the United States or Canada. (One or two had returned to Scandinavian countries.) I felt very out of place and very lonely. My father was very busy with his work as usual and I hardly saw him. He was working with young male Sudanese and Ugandan refugees who had fled to Kenya and ended up in Nairobi. He was running an outreach center downtown and was totally consumed with his work. Often he would bring refugees home for an evening meal and then would stay up for hours counseling them. At these times, I retreated to my bedroom.

My mother was at home some of the time, but she was recovering well and started to continue her own missionary work. This involved working in the office of a childcare center that was attached to the church they attended. I didn't have much to say to her anyway, as I was worried about my own situation. It is hard to make small talk when you are just eighteen, unmarried, and are worried that you might be pregnant. Couple this with the fact that I had no money, not a friend in sight, and was dreading getting the results of my "A" levels. I didn't know how long my parents would keep me in Kenya, had no means of transport and was 100 percent dependent on them. I needed to pass at least two "A" levels to secure a place in a teacher training college and I wasn't sure I had managed this. All of this was embarrassing for me. I arrived in England after graduating early from an American-style high school in Kenya with SAT scores of 92 percentile. Most universities would have been happy to enroll me at that time with those scores. I was too young so was advised to take a couple of years to complete "A" levels. What a different story it would be now!

To be truthful, it had been pretty hard to do any studying for my exams, even before I started going out with your father. My aunt's house was a typical three-bedroom, semi-detached, council house. It had a small galley kitchen, a front room and a living room downstairs. Upstairs there were three bedrooms and a small bathroom. My uncle and aunt slept in one bedroom, my two male cousins (ages nineteen and twenty-two) shared a very small bedroom and I shared with my two female cousins (ages fifteen and twenty-one). They shared a double bed and I had a single. My bed was the only part of the bedroom that was not three feet deep in discarded clothes. (There was so little cupboard space!) I had no desk and there was not even a table where I could sit and study or complete homework either upstairs or downstairs. Mostly I completed homework on my lap either sitting on my bed or on a chair in the front room. The house was generally a very noisy house; my uncle liked to watch the TV after he got in from work and my cousins liked to play music on the record player in the front room. It was also a very busy house as my cousins were very popular and their friends/girl-friends/boyfriends were always visiting. Added to that, three of them were in a gospel-singing group and regularly had practices at the house.

My Saturdays were spent working, first at a mail order company as a packer, then at a hairdresser as a general dogsbody (menial worker) and later for a large retail store in the food department. I needed to work, as my auntie and uncle could not afford to give me bus fares, buy me clothes, or give me dinner money or indeed any spending money. The money my parents sent them each month barely covered my board. After I started going out with your father, there was even less time and space in which to read, study or revise.

However, England and everything that had happened there seemed like a dream. I was very relieved to be away from your father, but he was writing to me and I was answering his letters. I didn't know what to do really. I knew that it would not be good to continue a relationship with him, but I was scared that I was pregnant and I didn't know whom to tell. Home was strange, as my sister was not there; she was by that time over in Canada about to start at Bible College. It was all really different; I was not used to living at home with my parents. Since the age of four, I had spent most of my time living in institutions. The only constant in my life before I went to England was my sister and she was absent.

Now I was eighteen and a very different person from the one who had left. My mother was not as ill as I had expected her to be. She had indeed had a bad fall and it had affected her neck and her balance somewhat, but I soon realized that my parents really wanted me back with them because they were worried about my relationship with your father. They had heard about it through my mother's relatives in Manchester. I am not really sure who had contacted them, but that is irrelevant now.

At first I was hopeful that my period was just late and that after I settled down in Kenya again, it would reappear. After all, my periods had stopped once before when I stopped eating regularly; maybe there was another explanation for the delay. I lived in hope. The days turned into weeks and still no period. I faked a heavy cold and asked my parents to take me to the doctor. My parents were puzzled when I asked to see the doctor by myself, but as I was eighteen, they let me go in alone. As soon as I got into the room, I was relieved to see that it was a woman doctor. I quickly explained the situation to her and she examined me. She told me I was indeed pregnant. I told her my circumstances and she urged me to tell my parents. She explained I had three options: keep you, have you adopted, or get a termination. She also explained that terminations were illegal in Kenya and that if that was my decision, I would need to go to a country where they were legal. I was totally shell shocked, even though it was as I had feared. I left the surgery in a daze, far too fearful to say anything to my parents.

By this time my parents had found me a part-time job, working as a secretary to an American man who was in Kenya with the United Nations. (Along with my A Levels, I had completed some courses in shorthand and typing.) My boss was from one of the southern states of the United States and none of the Kenyan secretaries could understand his accent so he had permission to hire a non-Kenyan.

I worked mornings and it was a nightmare. My father drove me to an office in downtown Nairobi and I started work at 8:00 a.m. I found the work difficult, more especially as I had acute morning sickness and for the first hour or so had to keep excusing myself to vomit in the toilets. I still had not managed to tell my parents my situation. The day came when I realized I would have to say something. My exam results had come through and I had a passed two "A" Levels and achieved a B grade and an E grade. My parents started talking about me returning to England to teacher training, but I realized that this would no longer be possible as I was pregnant. After much thought, I had decided to continue with my pregnancy. I was not sure if I would be able to keep you, but I thought that I could offer you up for adoption if I couldn't. I started thinking about names for you, I wondered if you were a boy or a girl. My idea at the time was that I would stay with my parents in Kenya until you were born. I hadn't really thought much beyond that. I knew I couldn't return to my auntie's as she had only arranged with my parents for me to live there for two years, much less continue to live there pregnant. The scandal would be enormous and the practicalities unimaginable. I had written to tell Colin that I was pregnant and to my surprise, he had sent me a very nice letter back saying we could get married quickly and I could go and live with him and his brothers. I knew I could not do this because of the way he had manipulated and abused me and I was by now far enough away to think more clearly. I realized that he would not change and I could not marry a man I feared and who forced me to do things against my will and made me feel dirty and used. So, my dear child, that was not an option; my life would have been a living hell and so would yours.

The day came when I braced myself to tell my parents. I came home from work in the early afternoon and went into my mother's bedroom to tell her that I was pregnant. She was lying on the bed reading a newspaper and having an afternoon rest. It is very common in Africa for people to have a rest after lunch in the heat of the day and it was my mother's habit. I started to chat to her about my day, but could not bring myself to tell her. In the end, I picked up her pen and whilst we were talking and I wrote on the edge of the newspaper, *"Mum, I am going to have a baby."* She started to cry and told me that she had suspected that something was wrong. I don't remember much else except that she was very worried about telling my dad. I agreed to tell him that evening at dinner and went to my room. My dad arrived home for dinner with three refugees in tow. We sat and ate dinner. I continued to sit at the table and listen to my dad talking to the three young refugee men. I kept hoping they would go so I could get a chance to speak to my father. In the end, I gave up waiting. I went to my mother in the kitchen and said that I would have to go to bed because I needed to get up for work in the morning and I was feeling very sick. I asked her to tell my dad for me. I knew he had to be told and now that my mum knew, it had to be that night. I think the refugees left after midnight and I didn't hear much after that.

In the morning, I got up and got dressed and went out to get some breakfast. My father was sitting at the table and as I approached the table his first words were, "How could you do this to us, Laura?" It was followed by, "I have been sitting here all night, praying, and I have decided that you must get rid of the baby." He then proceeded to ask me questions about how I got pregnant. He asked me how it had happened and how many times I had had sex.

"Once, it only happened once," I said, lying through my teeth, but I did not want to hurt him and I did not want him to think any more badly of me than he already did.

He proceeded to tell me that I had ruined his life and his Christian ministry and that the only solution was for me to tell no one about it and get an abortion. If I did not do this, my mum and he would have to quit the mission field in disgrace.

I could see that he was really upset, but at least it was out in the open now. I told him that I wanted to have the baby (you), but he said that that would not be possible and that it was unthinkable. He asked me how I could possibly look after a baby. I told him that I could stay with them until I had the baby and then I could put it up for adoption if they did not want me to live with them with the baby. I told him that abortion was illegal in Kenya. He said that I could not continue to live with them whilst pregnant and that they would not allow me to stay in Kenya and give birth to the baby, as it would ruin the work that they were doing there. I told him your father knew and he made me write a letter to him saying that I had made a mistake and in fact I was not pregnant at all. He forbade me to get in touch with your father again and told me that I was not to return to Manchester.

You have to realize that I was totally powerless. I had no money; nowhere to live, no one to talk to and the God of my early youth seemed very distant. I give my dad credit: on the few facts he knew he judged rightly in insisting that I was not to consider continuing a relationship with your father, but as for not allowing me to continue in the pregnancy and either keep you or put you up for adoption, I will never understand that part of it.

The time came to leave for work and my father drove me without speaking to me in the car. I have had some lonely days in my life, but that was one of the loneliest.

By the time I had finished work that day, my father had booked a flight to England. He left shortly afterwards, spending the next few weeks booking me into a private clinic just outside of London to have an abortion and finding me an alternative teacher training college.

The next couple of weeks were a blur. I don't remember speaking to my mother again about the fact that I was pregnant, but maybe I did. This was not the kind of things that were spoken of in our house. On the night before my mother left me in England at sixteen, she had attempted to speak to me about relationships between boys and girls. Her advice was that I should always stick with a group of friends and should never go off with a boy on my own. That, as far as I can remember, is the sum total of my personal sex education from my parents. My father never spoke to me about sex or relationships of any kind apart from when he found out I was pregnant.

I do remember that I resigned from my position as secretary and made the reason that I had decided to return to England to further my studies. I also remember that I had been working without pay whilst the man I worked for was sorting out financial transfers and setting up his office in Kenya. It was arranged that my boss would give my back pay to my parents, as by the time everything was sorted out I would be in the United Kingdom. The money never reached my hands and I had no choice as to how it was spent. My mother told me that it would go toward the cost of the flights and the abortion. What I am trying to tell you, my dear child, is that it seemed impossible at the time for me not to go along with my parents' plans.

To be honest, I do not even know how much the pay was or if it covered the costs. It is funny the things that you remember and the things that you forget. I do not recall anything about the flight or even being met at the airport in London by my father. I think it was Heathrow, but it may have been Gatwick. I do remember arriving at the abortion clinic, but I have no idea to this day where it was. My father drove me straight from the plane to the clinic. We walked in and I was led to a small room where there was a man behind a desk. After a brief conversation, where I was asked why I felt that I needed the abortion, I was asked to sign some papers. It was determined that my mental health would be damaged if I continued with the pregnancy. It was just a formality and did not constitute any kind of advice or counseling as to any course of action that was open to me apart from having an abortion. So you see, even at this stage I was not being given any options and was not pointed in any other direction apart from abortion. My father was standing behind me all the time and was directing my answers. Yet, deep down, I wanted to keep you. I did not want to go through with the abortion, but at the same time I just did not know how to do so, so I signed the papers. In a touch of normalcy, my father gave me a package containing a nightgown and some slippers. I truly think that from this point on, he blanked the whole thing from his conscious mind and treated it like a stay in hospital for a minor operation.

He left and I was led to an empty bed in a room with a few beds. There were women in all the other beds. No one spoke much; I guess we were all deep in thought, although I do recall speaking to a young woman on my left. We all knew why we were there so I guess there wasn't much else to say. It is not the kind of place that you make friends because it is the kind of place and kind of experience that you want to forget and put out of your mind as quickly as possible. I was hardly going to exchange phone numbers, and anyway, I did not have a phone number or even an address of my own.

My stay at the clinic lasted for a couple of days. I had a general anesthetic for the procedure, which was scary enough in itself. I cannot begin to fully describe how I felt during that time. Abandoned and alone with no way of communicating with anyone on the outside: afterwards you were gone and I was totally empty inside. I did not even know if you were a boy or a girl and I was not allowed to grieve for your passing. Physically I was drained and I was not prepared for the bleeding; it was like no period I have ever experienced. The name I had for you was Carly, because I kind of felt that you were a girl, but of course, I do not know.

My father arrived to pick me up in due course and when we were in the car, he informed me that I was on my way to an interview at a teacher training college in South London. Prior to my trip to Kenya, I had applied to a teacher training college in Manchester and been accepted depending on A level results, but my father had decided that I was not to take up that place. He had secured me an interview at a college in London. The term had already started, but they were prepared to interview me as they still had spaces on some courses and I had already been accepted at another college.

I remember sitting in the interview worried that I would get blood on the seat as I was bleeding so much. I don't remember much about the questions I was asked, but I was offered a place both on the course and in the halls of residence. It must have been a Friday as I was told to come back on the Sunday to move in and start lectures on the Monday. So dear child, I was taken straight from an abortion clinic to the college where I was to spend the next four years of my life. I have often wondered how my life would have been different if I had been allowed to have you. I certainly would not have started college that year. I may have put you up for adoption and then later you may have sought me out and we could have started a relationship as adults or I may have kept you. Knowing how I felt when my other babies were born, I do not think I would have been able to give you up. Although I was never given a due date for your birth, I worked it out that you would have been due in late March or early April. Every year I have imagined you at the age you would have been had you lived. Even to this day, I sometimes imagine you as a thirty-seven-year-old.

After the interview, my father took me to stay for the weekend with a close friend of the family in Kent. My father told me that she did not know what had happened to me and I was to pretend I had just arrived from Kenya and was to start college in London. So you can see that one lie has to be covered by many lies. One sin invariably leads to another. That night after she had gone to bed, he sat up with me and told me that I was never to speak about the "incident" as he called it again. I was never to write to my mother about it and I was never to tell anyone else what had happened. He forbade me to visit Manchester or to communicate with anyone there, particularly your father. My mother had written me a letter to read on the plane and I also had letters from your father that he made me bring to him. My auntie (this is what we called the family friend) had a fire going although it was only early October, and my father proceeded to burn the letters. My father made it clear to me that he would never talk about the "incident" again and that I must never mention it to my mother. I was in a state of shock and grief and bewilderment. My life had suddenly been turned upside-down again. The only friends I had in England were in Manchester and I was now banned from going there. Apart from the old Auntie we were staying with, I had no one I could turn to in London. I felt numb.

Two days later, my father drove me to the college. We got out of the car and my father helped me to take my one suitcase through the college grounds and along to the Halls of Residence where I had been assigned a room. The room itself was basic but comfortable. There was a single bed, a small desk, and a cupboard. Along the hallway there were toilets, sinks, and showering facilities. In a way, I was used to this kind of experience. I was a person who was used to living in an institution, as I had spent most of my life in hostels, children's homes, and boarding schools. I was used to packing and unpacking, I was used to the feeling of abandonment, but this time it was different. I felt really totally alone and rejected. I had no idea when I would see my father or mother again and my sister was now in Canada. I had always had her there with me at boarding schools and even though we did not always get along, it was somehow comforting to have someone else in the family sharing my experience. I was now not allowed to go and see all the family and friends I had come to know in Manchester. I did not even want to go back there because I did not want to see your father. I had no idea what I would say to him and was in fact very afraid that if he found out where I was that he would come looking for me. I can't actually explain fully how I felt. It was as if I was in a very bad dream and soon I would wake up and find out that none of the bad stuff had happened.

My father did not stay very long and I walked back with him to the car to say goodbye. He was flying back to Nairobi the next day to rejoin my mother. He had to get back in time for a planned celebration, as it was their twenty-fifth wedding anniversary. It all seemed very surreal to me; life was going on as if nothing had happened. My father never made mention of the event that ended your life ever again, even up to his death nineteen years later.

I was still bleeding quite heavily, but having to pretend that this was just a normal goodbye, kind of like a "see you later." My father gave me a Bible and inside he had written the date and the words "*Congratulations on passing your "A" Levels and entering college. Love, Mummy and Daddy.*"

It was his attempt at normalcy and I do still have the Bible so it must have meant something to me at the time. I waved goodbye to him as he drove away and walked slowly back to my new room. A new chapter in my life was starting as your life had ended. Shortly afterwards, I bought some cigarettes and started to smoke. They were my constant companions for the next twenty-five years along with a few other unwanted friends, namely: guilt, bitterness, and shame.

Love,

Your mother

xxxx

LETTER 2

Hope

Dear child,

As I write this, I am sitting waiting for one of your sisters. She is at a doctor's appointment. On the wall is a poster and on the poster is a picture of a beautiful waterfall. Underneath the picture are the words: *Turn your scars into stars.*

This is what I have tried to do with the scars in my life and losing you is one of those scars. I am trying to make it into a star by writing about it and sharing my experience with others.

As you know from my first letter, your maternal grandparents were missionaries in Africa and I was brought up there. I was brought up knowing the Bible and to believe that there was a God and that he cared for me. Most of the time, I implicitly believed everything I was taught. I certainly believed that Jesus was God and that he came to earth with a purpose and that purpose was to save mankind from their sin. I believed that the only way to heaven was through belief in Jesus, but somewhere along the way I got lost and confused. This, I think, is because there also seemed to be a lot of rules involved, some of which I understood as being moral and right, and some that I did not really understand or know why they were wrong. So for example, I understood that it is wrong to steal, to murder, and to lie, but some of the rules just did not make sense to me. I could not understand why, as a girl, it was wrong for me to wear shorts or trousers, or why at times I was not allowed to cut my hair.

Looking back, I can see that the rules that made sense were the ones that were linked to the Ten Commandments and the ones that did not make sense were linked to traditions, expectations, and interpretations of the Bible. To be honest, most of the time, I just accepted the rules and obeyed them to the best of my ability. I did not like getting into trouble and avoided confrontation. I actually don't remember ever really defying my parents or speaking back to them or even questioning any of their rules. I think that this is partly why, although it was not what I wanted, I went along with the abortion that they planned. I was used to obeying them and so I obeyed. At the time, I could not see any other way without their help. I felt trapped.

I now know that I had a choice. I still feel that I was "forced" to have an abortion and certainly at the time no other option was presented to me, but I also accept that even at the clinic I could have said "no," and that it is never too late to change your mind about these things. I do not know what would have then happened, whether my parents would have disowned me and abandoned me, whether I would have been surreptitiously dumped with my suitcase on the streets of London to make my own way in life or whether they would have softened and reconsidered their position. There are endless possibilities and permutations; certainly my life would have been very different, but it was not to be. I did not stand up to them. Once I realized (more than twenty-five years later) that by not standing up against them, I had chosen to go along with their decision, I was then able to accept responsibility for my action. I was then able to accept God's forgiveness for my action and to go on to forgive my parents for their actions. It was indeed a wonderful release. I felt the bitterness that I had harbored melt away. For years, I had blamed them for the abortion and I had never looked beyond what I considered to be their guilt. I had never examined my own actions and motives; I had never seen my own weakness and culpability.

So what was it that brought this about? What was it that transformed my thinking about this incident and my life in general? It was an acceptance of Jesus as *my* Savior. My eyes were opened to the reality of a God who cared enough about me to send his son Jesus to die for me. I realized that being a follower of Jesus Christ was not a list of rules and regulations, not a list of do's and don'ts, but entering into a relationship with the one true living God. I realized that I had spent a lot of my life looking to other people and blaming them when things went wrong, instead of looking to God for my strength and salvation.

I spent a lot of my childhood apart from my parents and when I went to do my Teacher Training after I lost you, I found out that statistically I was "maternally deprived" as I had been separated from my mother before the age of four to live in a children's' hostel. I am sure that this has had a bearing on the way I have lived my life and in particular on the way I have parented my own children. As for you, my dear child, I did not get the chance to parent you, but again know that I loved you and that I truly believe that we will meet up again someday. This is part of my hope.

So in my despair, hope came, but it took a long time: twenty-five-and-a-half years, two marriages, two more births, a miscarriage, and a mental breakdown to be exact. It's more if you consider that after I found hope, it then took me a further twelve months to be truly reconciled to my own mother and to come to terms with what I did to you and to feel forgiven and even more when you add on the ten years, one more miscarriage and one more birth, it has taken me since then to write this letter. So where do I get the hope of seeing you again? I get this hope from the Bible. One day I was reading 2 Samuel chapter twelve. In verse 23 of this chapter, King David tells his servants that he has stopped mourning now that his sick child is dead. He writes: "But now he has died: why should I fast? Can I bring him back again? I will go to him, but he will not return to me."

It was when I read this verse that I realized that although I could never bring you back, I will go to be with you, when I eventually die. I believe this because like King David, I believe that I will go to be with God when I die and that you are already there. So there it is; finally I have resolution, and I have hope. We will spend eternity together. What I did was wrong, but I am forgiven. Death is not the end; eternity is waiting.

There are some people who will think I am deluded, and others to whom this may give the same hope. There are debates about when life starts. Some say that life starts only when a baby is born and takes its first breath and some like me believe that life starts at conception. So for me, dear child, you were a human life from the moment of your conception. There are many references in the Bible to babies in the womb. The one I find most beautiful and uplifting is in Psalm 139. This is a Psalm of David. From verse 13, it reads:

For you formed my inward parts;

You wove me in my mother's womb.

I will give thanks to You, for I am fearfully and wonderfully made;

Wonderful are your works,

And my soul knows it very well.

My frame was not hidden from You,

When I was made in secret,

And skillfully wrought in the depths of the earth;

Your eyes have seen my unformed substance;

And in Your book were all written

The days that were ordained for me,

When as yet there was not one of them.

This shows me that God knows us when we are still unborn and in our mother's womb. This also shows me that we are therefore a human life whilst still in the womb. This is why I believe, dear child, that you were a human life and now have a heavenly life.

My reconciliation with my own mother was sweet and I love her dearly. This again came about when I was reading the Bible, this time a very well known passage, known and loved by many, which suddenly came alive for me. It is the third verse of Psalm 23.

He restores my soul;

He guides me in the paths of righteousness

For his name's sake.

It doesn't say that God might restore my soul; it says that God restores my soul and that he guides or leads me in the paths of righteousness. I knew that as God had forgiven me so now my soul was restored and I was able—indeed obligated—to forgive others. To put it simply, God guided me to forgive my mother and to tell her so. It also made me ask for her forgiveness for my part in the grief I had caused her and my father by getting pregnant. Again, I did this through writing her a letter. I must be the kind of person who finds it easier to express my inner feelings in writing rather than through speech. I can think the words, but sometimes I cannot actually say them in person. I was sorry that I could not forgive my father in person as he passed away before hope came to me, but God knows my heart and knows that I have forgiven him also. Dear child, this forgiveness has been the most wonderful thing.

I remember once I was in an open AA meeting, and one of the people in the group was talking about un-forgiveness and resentment. They likened harboring un-forgiveness and resentment in oneself to getting a deadly poison, pouring it into a glass for another person, but then drinking it yourself. This is what I think I had been doing for years. No wonder I ended up having a breakdown. Life is hard and we humans need to learn to let some things go. I was happy to let go of the guilt, bitterness, and shame that I had felt since my abortion and when your youngest brother was conceived, I was also able to get rid of the cigarette addiction that had dogged me for so many years. My new companions are faith, hope, and love.

Love,

Your Mother

xxxx

2

To the Children of My First Marriage

LETTER 1

A Boy Is Born

Daniel, Daniel, Daniel, my dearest Daniel,

Your birth was a completely and utterly life-changing event for me: agony coupled with amazement. The birth itself was one of the most exhilarating experiences in my life. I had no idea at all what to expect. I had no friends who had babies, I had never lived in a house with babies, and nobody had ever spoken to me about childbirth apart from the midwives at the hospital. I had no interest in other people's babies. After I lost my first unborn child, I had done my best not to think about babies.

During my pregnancy, I had not been able to attend any of the antenatal classes due to the fact that I worked full time until the day before you were due. I guess everyone just expected me to know all about it. I mean I knew it was going to be painful; I just didn't know how painful. I knew life was going to be different afterwards; I just didn't know how different. I had no idea how it would change the way I felt about life so completely. I did not know how my body would suddenly belong to someone else and how completely I would be bowled over by this baby of mine. The first time I walked down the street after you were born, I had new eyes. I looked at every mother and every child with utter amazement. I just could not believe that these women had been through what I had just been through. Suddenly, I had great admiration for all women everywhere, and if they had more than one child, well, there were no words to express how much I admired them. They had actually

21

gone through what I had just gone through and had the guts to do it again!

The birth itself was nothing at all like I expected. On all the movies I ever watched, it seemed to be all over and done within ten minutes and the end result was a beautiful clean baby all wrapped up, who automatically nestled into his or her mother's arms. The mother, of course, looked slightly disheveled, but still beautiful with makeup intact. I, on the other hand, went into labor on Wednesday and you arrived on Friday! I was utterly exhausted when you were born and more than a little disheveled. Your dad gave up waiting to celebrate your birth and went out drinking with his best mate during the labor. He was there for your actual birth, but missed most of the warm up. I remember feeling very lonely and scared during the labor and utter relief when you finally arrived. I did not know whether you were going to be a boy or a girl, but I was happy to have either. Your dad and I had decided that if you were a boy, he would choose your name and if you were a girl, I would choose your name. Before you were born, he gave me a list of boy's names that he liked and I picked one of them. When you were born, he was so excited that you were a boy. I was just happy that you had arrived and that you were healthy and beautiful. Those first few days are a bit of a blur. I didn't sleep and my emotions were all over the place. At times I was ecstatic and at others dejected. You made me ecstatic; I could not believe I had produced anything so wonderful. On the other hand, my inexperience and lack of family support made me feel dejected. I was worried about how I was going to cope with a new baby, an unreliable, drinking husband, and my work.

My own parents were by this time living in England, having retired from their work in Africa, but they did not come to see us in hospital even though I was there for ten days. I felt abandoned by them yet again. Some of the days and nights, we had no visitors at all. I pulled the curtains around my hospital bed during visiting hours so that other people wouldn't look at us. Looking back, I think that your paternal grandparents assumed that your dad was visiting us every evening after work when in fact he was out drinking to celebrate your birth. The thing about drinkers is that any occasion is an excuse to drink. They drink if it's sunny, they drink if it's wet, they drink if they get a job, and they drink if they lose a job, they drink at a funeral, they drink at a birth, and even if there is no occasion, they drink.

As for you, my Daniel, you captivated my every waking and sleeping thoughts—well, not that much sleeping went on I must admit! One of the things I had expected was that a baby would sleep a lot. You made me aware that this was a mere illusion right from the outset. Daytime sleeps were completely off your list of "to dos" and nighttime sleeps didn't appeal to you much either. After I left hospital, I have many memories of pacing up and down our small living room trying to rock you to sleep in my arms in the small hours of the night. You didn't like it when I sat down and started to scream if I did so. You didn't like it if I put you in a baby rocking chair and started to scream if I did so. You didn't like being in anything that restrained you apart from my arms. When I spoke to the midwife about your lack of sleep and your dislike of being put down, she assured me it was a sign of your intelligence and that I should worry if you were listless and took no interest in life.

Don't think it was all just tiring, because you need to remember that I was totally besotted by you. I loved you more than I had ever loved anyone or anything. I could not believe the emotions that you aroused in me. There was finally some healing after losing my first unborn child ten years earlier. It was as if my body had been waiting for a baby for ten years and you had finally arrived. This had not been a conscious yearning, rather a subconscious yearning. It changed the way I looked at other people. It changed the way I felt when watching the news, especially if there was a disaster of any kind that involved children. I would openly weep. For so many years, all my feelings had been kept under tight control. I did not like to show my emotions to others. Your every breath, your every sound, and your every movement also fascinated me. I was scared sometimes when I was holding you that I would drop you. When I was first walking out of the hospital ten days after walking in, in labor, I could not believe that they were actually allowing me to leave with you in my arms. I had been taught how to feed, change, and bathe you in the hospital, but there had always been someone on hand to give advice or to help; now it was just going to be me. Scary!

When you were born, I was nearly twenty-eight years old and had been married to your father for four-and-a-half years. We were living in a two bedroom flat in South East London. It was part of an old terraced house, probably Victorian that had been converted into two flats. We lived downstairs, which meant we had access to the small back garden.

When I discovered I was pregnant, I was totally bowled over. It was entirely unexpected although looking back I don't know why—after all, I was married! Really, I guess I was surprised because I had been taking contraception, which seemed to have worked pretty well for years. At the time of your conception, I had decided to change my method of contraception and it was during this changeover period that you were conceived. Although at the time I believed I had taken all the necessary precautions to ensure that I would not get pregnant, this was obviously not the case.

You might well wonder why I would not want to get pregnant; after all, I was approaching five years into a marriage and getting quite old to have a first baby. Well, the reason was that I realized my marriage was very fragile. I was not sure that your dad loved me. I thought that he had a drinking problem and he had already left me once and tried to end the marriage just two months before I discovered I was pregnant. Living in London was very expensive and although your dad was earning quite a decent wage at the time, as a painting and decorating subcontractor, we never seemed to see much of his money, as it all seemed to disappear. My wage as a teacher paid all the bills and we were struggling to make ends meet. I was stuck in a bit of a rut in my job and had applied for a secondment from my regular teaching job, to study the use of computers in education. This would involve a year out doing full-time study at Kings College that was part of the University of London. I was really excited to have been accepted on the course and looking forward to the opportunity to study again. So being pregnant was going to complicate things a little. Once I found out I was pregnant, I made enquiries to see if I could start the course, have a maternity leave, and then resume the course a year later. At the time, teachers in the ILEA (Inner London Education Authority) where I worked were entitled to a year's maternity leave (some paid, some unpaid). I was told that basically it was "now or never." They weren't sure that the course would run a second time so if I wanted to continue, I would have to complete the course in the year—pregnant or not.

This left me in a quandary. Having an abortion was completely out of the question. The first one had devastated me completely and I still grieved the baby I had lost so that was not part of my dilemma. The dilemma was whether or not to take up the opportunity to study for a year whilst being pregnant. I spoke to my doctor who very wisely told me that pregnancy was not an illness, but a natural part of life. She encouraged me to continue with my plans for as long as I could; if I gave up on the study because of being pregnant I might later resent the child I was carrying. She assured me that she would monitor my health and if she thought it was suffering, she would advise me to leave the course.

As it happened, I stayed on the course until the day before you were due, which actually fell on the Easter break. The other students had a six-week study leave; I had a baby—you—and returned to the university six weeks after you were born and only one week after the other students. I passed the course and even managed the one-day-a-week placement in a school. I breastfed you fully until I returned to the University, and then partially for a few months. I can remember stuffing breast pads down my bra like there was no tomorrow, because initially, I leaked so much breast milk during the day. Leaving such a tiny baby in the care of someone else whilst I finished the course was one of the hardest things I have ever had to do. You were a part of me; I thought about you all day and couldn't wait to pick you up in the evenings. You were looked after by your grandparents (on your dad's side) for three days a week and by a friend of a friend of mine who had also had a new baby for the other two days. Although your dad was a drinker, alcohol had not completely taken over his life at the time of your birth. In those early days, he took part in all aspects of your care: he changed your nappy, he bathed you, he dressed you, he cuddled you, and he even sang to you. When I started to wean you from breast milk, he also fed you from time to time. He decorated the second bedroom in our flat for you and when he wasn't out drinking was very attentive to you. In fact, he knew more about babies than I did. As you know, he is the oldest of four children and your uncle was born when your dad was sixteen so he was quite used to having a baby in the house. He was very aware of potential dangers in the home and was very safety conscious as far as you were concerned; he just wasn't there enough.

After I had you, Daniel, I could never imagine a life without you. You were the most amazing baby in the whole world. I delighted in every milestone you made. By nine and a half months, you were able get up and stand unaided and by ten months you were walking.

It was at this time that your father and I decided to move away from London. It was very expensive and we were finding it hard to make ends meet. Your dad seemed to be drinking more and more, but now having a baby, I was not able to go out with him in the evening so I do not really know how much he was drinking. At that time, he usually went to the pub. Even when we went out as a little family during the day at the weekend, we always seemed to end up in a pub. Your dad became expert at finding pubs where we were allowed to take in a baby. Your dad told me that he was unhappy in his job and that he was sorry he had left school at sixteen. He wanted to get a degree so that he could have better job opportunities. I could understand him wanting to better himself and thought that if he was able to achieve this, it would make him happy and he would then drink less. I was still very much a novice at this drinking game. My parents had brought me up as teetotal and I had never really seen anyone drink alcohol sensibly. I started to drink myself whilst at teacher training college and looking back, I have to say that most people I knew at college drank to excess, but of course, I did not really know any different way of drinking. I thought all people who drank had ten pints or more in an evening so did not think that your dad's drinking was that unusual when we were going out, but being married to a drinker was a different story. This was not Friday night drinking; this was every day drinking. This was being unable to stay at home for one evening without a trip to the pub, kind of drinking. This was spending money on drink when we didn't have enough money for bills. This was not intending to go out for a drink, but having to go anyway.

So I guess, Daniel, that it was at this point that I truly realized that alcohol was becoming the third "person" in my marriage. However, I actually thought that if your dad felt more fulfilled in his career/work life, he would not feel the need for alcohol and we would then be happy. We realized that he could not go to college in London, as it was too expensive for us to continue to live there on one wage. Your dad applied for places at teacher training colleges in the north of England and was accepted provisionally at two of them as a mature student. I resigned my job in London, which I had returned to after my year at the University of London. The plan was for me to get work initially as a supply teacher and from that position to move into full-time work. Your dad would look after you whilst I worked and would prepare to start college in September.

Everything seemed to be falling into place as we made our plans. My parents were living in Stoke-on-Trent, but were planning on returning to Africa for a year to work in Zambia as relief missionaries. This meant that their house would be vacant and they needed to rent it out. It was agreed that we would live in their house and rent it from them whilst they were away. So we sold our little flat and moved.

Surprise, surprise, the move did not dissipate your father's drinking as I had hoped, but I was still optimistic that he would stop drinking once he actually started his studies and was on his road to fulfillment. I got work as a supply teacher and spent one term teaching in a few schools in the area. At the time, I did not have a driving license and not being able to drive proved a problem, as there was not the public transport that I was used to in London, so I took up driving lessons. During this time, Daniel, your dad stayed at home and looked after you. Whilst I was at work, he fed you, played with you, changed your nappy and was a real dad to you. In the evenings, he drank almost from the moment I returned from work. After the move, he had started drinking in the house more and more as he had no drinking mates and didn't like the local pub.

Then the surprise bombshell hit: I was pregnant again. The sole breadwinner of the family, about to support her husband through college was having another baby. We were, however, happy that I was pregnant.

"It's not good for a child to be the only one," your dad said.

For me it was, of course, another reason that your dad would have to stop drinking. I mean you can't carry on drinking when there are two little mouths to feed and clothe, can you? I was happy that the new baby would be close in age to you as my sister and I are close in age and it just seemed right somehow. So, Daniel, although there were definitely storm clouds brewing big time on the horizon of my marriage, your birth was a defining and healing moment in my life and you were born to parents who loved you. This is what you need to know.

Love,

Mum

xxxx

LETTER 2

A Girl Is Born

Dear Sally,

The year was 1987. On the day you were born, Britain had just experienced severe stormy weather with a mini-hurricane and gale force winds causing havoc in much of the south. I was living near my parents' house in Stoke-on-Trent where your dad and I had moved only three months earlier. For six months prior to that, we had been living in Nana and Granddad's house in Stoke. Your dad is a Londoner through and through, as you know, but we had ended up in the north of England for financial reasons and because your dad wanted to go to University as a mature student. The plan was that I would support him through college. I know that you know now that not everything in life goes according to plan; in fact, most things don't!

When we first moved up to Stoke, my mum and dad had not yet gone back to Congo, so as a parting gift they offered to look after Daniel whilst your dad and I had a weekend to ourselves. It was a much-needed break. We had not been getting on very well and since Daniel was born, I had not seen much of your dad in the evenings as he went out drinking every night. I was working full time in a very demanding teaching job and basically just crossing paths with your dad after I arrived home from picking up Daniel from your grandma's. Your dad would eat, spend a little time with Daniel, help with the bathing, feeding, and getting to sleep and then leave. Daniel was not a good sleeper, so often after your dad returned home, I would then be up with him for hours in the night before getting ready for work the next morning. Enough about Daniel—this is about you!

For the weekend away, we chose Stratford-upon-Avon as it was relatively close and I wanted to see Shakespeare country. It was a good weekend and your dad did not drink as much as usual. This was, I believe, when you were conceived and the dates tie in to your birth. I am telling you this because I want you to know that you were conceived during a pleasant holiday weekend away. I am telling you this, Sally, because a lot of what has happened since has not been pleasant; there has been pain and rejection so it is important for you to know that I believe you were conceived at this time.

You are now twenty-three and just yesterday, we were having a talk together and you were able to recall a rare time when your dad sat down and talked to you about relationships and about what real men look for in a woman. You told me that during that talk your dad made you feel good about yourself. I think you were about fourteen or fifteen at the time and you were visiting him in London. It is important for you to remember the good things about your dad and not just the bad.

Back to the night of your birth (we mothers just love to talk about our birthing experiences!) Nana had come over from Congo to be with me so she could see the new baby. I must have finally been able to express my distress that she had not come to see me when Daniel was born, whilst on the other hand twice travelling out to Kenya to be with my sister, Aunty Lina, when she had her two boys. She had arrived just before you were due, but you were already two weeks late on this night and she was getting worried that she would have to go back to Congo without ever seeing you. Your dad had started college and I was not seeing very much of him at all. He was out a lot in the evenings and your "London" family had all moved up north to the same area as us. Some of the time, he would go out with his sisters, sometimes with people from college. On other occasions, he would go out with his best friend from London, who by this time was living with my cousin in Manchester and would come down for dinking sessions. I think that Nana, my mum, was getting a little worried so she offered to babysit Daniel whilst your dad and I went out together.

It was a Friday night and your dad took me to a little pub (no surprises there then!). It was at the end of the high street in the small town where we were living. There were some college mates of his in the pub and we sat with them. I noticed two girls in particular that he seemed very friendly with and they also knew your Auntie Patricia and had been out with her and dad. At the time, I did not think much of it, being a little preoccupied at forty-two weeks pregnant. After pub closing time, we decided to cross the road and go to the Chinese take-away just across the road. I remember that it was quite busy, as the pub clientele had just basically "fallen" out of the pub and into the take-away. We placed our order and were standing waiting. Suddenly, I had a very strange sensation; I felt a gushing of water down the inside of my legs. There was no pain, just the water. Instantly I realized that my labor had begun, this time with my waters breaking. I told your dad, but at the same time our order was up so he collected the order and then drove us home. (Yes, I know I have always told you not to get in cars with people, who have been drinking, but your dad regularly drank and then drove and I didn't really have an option that night.) It is because of my experiences with your dad that I feel so strongly about it now. Anyway, back to the story: I continued to feel wet down below and my clothes were by this time soaking. When I got home, I told my mum what had happened and she being a midwife told me to ring the hospital and tell them I was coming in immediately. I rang the hospital and they confirmed that I should come in straight away even though I had no labor pains as yet. So excitement reigned. I quickly changed, grabbed my overnight bag (that had been packed for a couple of months) and my hospital notes, my mum gave me some towels to sit on in the car, and off we went. I was very nervous about your dad driving; he had been drinking heavily and the hospital was a thirty-minute drive away, but I didn't have enough money for a taxi.

The drive was okay and he got me there safely. By this time, the labor pains had started and I was admitted straight away to the labor ward. I had had it written in capital letters on the front page of my notes that I wanted an epidural. (I had been in labor for forty-two hours with Daniel and had thought I was dying, the pain was so extreme.) When I had discovered I was pregnant again, I was determined to have as little pain as possible. However, we are talking the North Staffs hospital here, back in the eighties, and they told me that the anesthetists did not work at night so I was rooked! Basically, unless it looked like I was dying, they were not going to call an anesthetist in! So much for birth preferences in the not-so-sunny Stoke!

You must have known that I could not take the pain, as you came out sweetly within six hours and I managed the pain with gas pethadin. Your dad stayed for the birth and held my hand. He did not keep disappearing as he had when Daniel was born; I guess that was because you didn't take forty-two hours and he was already well tanked up!

I was absolutely overjoyed that you were a girl. Perfect: I now had a boy and a girl. I was so blessed. I was over the moon. You were not quite as big as Daniel at eight pounds, six ounces; he had been just less than nine pounds, but was a very healthy weight, yet again proving all the experts wrong. They had been telling me all along that you were going to be a very small baby. You also decided to turn and come out headfirst as up until this point your head had not properly engaged and you had been in a breech position until a few days earlier. The name I had decided upon for a girl was Siobhan, but as I gazed lovingly at your little face it just somehow did not seem right so you were just baby Moran for a few hours whilst I tried to think of another name. (Your dad and I had agreed that I could name the baby if it was a girl, so it was up to me.)

After the birth, it seemed that all was not well with me. I felt very dizzy and light headed. I knew that you were okay and I could see you in a little see-through crib on the right of the bed, but I felt very weak. Your dad had gone back home, but I was still in the labor ward. I was vaguely aware that nurses were coming and going and peering at my private parts. They told me that the placenta had not followed you, as it should have and that I was losing a lot of blood—flooding, in fact. They strapped up my legs in stirrups and went in search of a doctor, leaving the door open onto the corridor. Oh the shame of it—I felt completely humiliated! My private parts, which were oozing blood, were completely on display to any random person who cared to walk by and look in! Yet, I was too weak to call out or say anything.

After what seemed an eon of time, a nurse came back with a doctor, who quickly examined me and then told me he was going to deliver the placenta with forceps, which he did. By this time, I was weeping and this got to him for some reason because I heard him ask the nurse why I was crying, after all I had had a completely healthy baby. He obviously had not done the course on bedside manners! The nurse put him right for which I was grateful, as I could not speak. Some bloods arrived as they had been contemplating a blood transfusion, but it appeared the hemorrhaging had stopped so they decided against the transfusion. I was still very weak so they put me in a recovery ward for a few hours. As I lay in the ward, all I could think about was finding a new name for you, my sweetheart. As I lay gazing at your by now sleeping form, the name Sally just popped into my head from nowhere and would not go away. It was not a name I had ever even contemplated before, but it somehow fit, so that, my dear, is how you got your name. Later in the day, we were moved to the maternity ward, but I was told not to get out of bed. My blood pressure was extremely low and I was weak and nauseous. I also could not do a wee and had to have a catheter. In order to move the placenta, the doctor had cut me down below and I was very sore and nothing felt right.

I kept looking at you in the plastic crib beside the bed and was so happy that you were a girl and that you were healthy. Perfect, I thought, a boy and a girl. I could not have wished for better. The next couple of days passed in a haze because I really was not very well at all. I remember that your dad's parents visited once and that your dad brought Nana and Daniel to see me the next day. I still could not get out of bed or lift you out of your crib. On the fourth day, after the catheter was removed and I was being assisted to walk to the toilet, your dad came up to the hospital to collect us. The staff tried to persuade him to leave me in hospital, but he said he wanted us home. They explained to him that I was still very weak and needed to be in hospital. He said that he would look after me when I got home. Where we lived was only about a thirty-minute drive away from the hospital and sure enough there was a beef stew waiting for me to eat, which your dad had cooked. We ate the meal and then your dad said that he was going out for an hour.

He did not return for a week. When he did return, it was only to have a shower and collect some clothes. He told me that he did not love me and that he wanted a divorce. I was totally shell shocked. Nana had been visiting us, but was due to go back to Africa where my dad was critically ill. They had gone back to work there in their retirement, but my mum had come back because she wanted to be there when you were born. I guess she realized how upset I had been that they ignored me when Daniel was born. I was totally desperate. Here I was stuck in some village near Stoke-on-Trent where I had no friends, no job, no family, a new baby, a very active toddler, and my husband had just abandoned us. Although he was a drinker, I was not expecting to be abandoned in this way.

My mother went back to Africa and my whole world seemed to crumble. I could not eat and was losing weight. I could not sleep and was constantly on the verge of tears. One of the hardest things was that I had no way of getting hold of your dad and had no idea where he was. He was receiving a student grant directly and I was on state maternity benefit, which was very meager. So to top it all, I had little or no money. I had been using disposable nappies for Daniel, but could no longer afford them so I also remember that the house was full of terry nappies, either being soaked or washed or on the line drying. After another week or so, I found out where your dad was staying and one night I collected all his clothes and personal belongings and put them into bin bags. An old friend from college days had come to visit me from Liverpool and she minded you and Daniel whilst I went and dumped all the bin bags outside the room your dad was renting. I had also taken the liberty of cutting up a number of our wedding photos and throwing the cut up pictures on top of the bags. So you see, I was a little deranged myself to say the least.

You slept a lot of the day at first, but were awake for most of the night in the first few weeks. This time, there was no one there to help me change, bathe, or rock the new baby to sleep and I also had Daniel who was extremely active. He had been walking since he was ten months old and he was in constant motion, into absolutely everything. Somehow I got through the next couple of months; I joined the local Labor Party and made a few friends that way. One night, I got a babysitter and went to a Labor Party meeting. Afterwards, I was invited out to the pub and I went along determined to try to make some friends and connections, as I had none. Lo and behold, whilst sitting there in the pub, your dad walked in as bold as brass with a couple of other college students. I recognized them as being the two girls we had sat with the night you were born. I literally froze to the spot. After what seemed like an eternity, but was probably only a minute, I explained the situation to my new friends and said that I would have to leave; they persuaded me to stay. Their reasoning was that I was there first and that if anyone should be uncomfortable it was not me, but him. To my surprise, they were right and after only a couple of minutes he left.

Months later, they told me that one of my new friends was the sister of the landlady of the pub and that your dad was well known there. He regularly came in with one of the girls with whom he was having an affair. It was a relatively small town and he was not well liked, as they all knew that he was married and that his wife had just had a baby. It also turned out that one of the people I was out with was a lecturer at the college and was your dad's history tutor. So there I was thinking I was walking around the village incognito, but in fact quite a few people knew my situation. Some of the friends I met that night remained my friends for years to come.

So you can see that your birth, although greatly anticipated and received with great joy, also came in a time of great anguish for me. It was weird; something had happened when I was six months pregnant with you that had really scared me and had caused me to shut down emotionally, but I still had this idea that marriage is forever, for better or worse, and that separation or divorce was not right. I am not sure whether I should include this incident because it was not typical of your dad, but it is relevant because his violence did surface on a few other occasions. I am not saying that your dad was a wife beater, but there were a couple of occasions in our ten years together that he used physical violence against me. Looking back, I recognize that he abused me a lot emotionally by constantly telling me I was useless, but he did not beat me up. I had believed that the cause of all my marriage troubles was alcohol and that one day your dad would see sense and stop drinking. Maybe when he finished his degree and got a different kind of job he would feel happier with his life and not need to drink—or so I thought. I also strongly believed that violence was wrong. I was not stupid and I knew all about domestic violence, particularly against women, but sometimes when you are in a situation, you can't see the wood for the trees. I had always believed, since my experience with the knife and my first boyfriend that at the first sign of violence in any relationship, I would run and that it would be right to do so. I would counsel any girl or woman to do the same, then and now.

However, when I was six months pregnant with you, your dad pushed me, shook me and punched me in the stomach in an angry encounter at the side of the road. He was very drunk and had rung me to come and pick him up, which I had done. I had only just passed my driving test and was not used to being in charge of a car. On the way home, the car broke down (ran out of petrol) and when we got out to ring the RAC from a phone box (no mobile phones in those days) the keys got locked in the car. Your dad blamed me and that is when he pushed, shook, and punched me, at the same time screaming abuse. I was holding Daniel in my arms and passers by were staring, but doing nothing. He then ran off leaving me to sort out the car, which of course, I did. Later when the drink wore off, he came home sobbing and begging me to forgive him. I understand now that this is often a pattern with abusive men, but at the time I thought he was sorry; nevertheless something inside of me snapped. That day I took off my wedding and engagement rings and I never wore them again.

Some of this stuff you know because over the years I have told you, but some of it is news to you. I always tell everyone that you were the perfect baby and you were. After the first few weeks of settling into a routine, you just slept, ate, giggled, played, and slept. You were the most content of all my babies, always giggling and smiling and so, so content. I remember that in the evening, I would bath you first, dry you, dress you in your nightclothes, and put you in your cot whilst I bathed Daniel. By the time I finished bathing Daniel, you would be fast asleep in your cot and that would be you until the next morning. So sweet!

Of course, the events surrounding your first few years do not end here. Your dad came crawling back when you were a couple of months old and I agreed to have him back. He had denied having an affair, but later had to admit to it. The affair and the lies continued to destroy our marriage. He continued to drink and I joined an organization called Al Anon, which helped me through the next fifteen years of my life. He flunked the first year of college because of his drinking. (He was so hung over on the morning of one of his exams that he did not attend the exam and the same happened on the date of the make-up exam.) So that whole venture had been a waste of time. He got a few casual jobs and was constantly on at me to refinance our house to set up a business with him. In the meantime, I had to return to work when you were three months old, as we had no money.

At first, your dad's parents who had moved up north, too, looked after you and Daniel whilst I went to work, but it soon proved too much for them, as they were also caring for their own youngest son and two other grandchildren that were living with them. Your next caretaker was a child minder called Diane, but when she became ill, I decided to send you both to nursery whilst I worked. Although your dad was not working all of the time, he was in no fit state to look after you.

So I plodded on, trying to make my marriage work and trying to keep a roof over our heads by working. Once again, your dad was drinking our money away and things were not getting any better.

I left him once, but returned when he made lots of promises to stop drinking. He did not keep the promises. However, when you were two and a half, and I had threatened to leave him again, he did give up drinking for a while. He was awful to live with, very aggressive and argumentative and all the time I felt like he was spoiling for a drink, just seeking that argument that could give him the "right" to go out and get drunk. We moved to a better house and I hoped yet again that this would make him happy, but it did not.

Sadly what this meant for you was that there was too much going on in your dad's life for him to truly bond to you. I don't know if it is because you were a girl, or some other reason, but he just never was the same with you as he was with Daniel. It may be that as the years went by, you reminded him of me and as he was angry with me so he was angry with you. Only your dad can tell you that. I, on the other hand, felt very close to you both and loved my little girl to death. You were the apple of my eye and just so sweet and beautiful.

Love,

Mum

xxxx

LETTER 3

Through Separation and Divorce

Dear Daniel and Sally,

This is a letter that I feel that you two can share. It is about shared times and shared experiences. It is about the time that we were a threesome. This was a difficult, but very precious time for us.

It is hard for me to write about this, even years later. I was brought up to believe that marriage was for life and that divorce was wrong. If you made a promise you should keep it and I had certainly made some promises to your dad when I married him. I had promised that I would stay with him "in sickness and in health," and alcoholism is regarded as an illness by some people, so theoretically, I should have stayed with your dad or I was a liar. I guess I just could not hack it any longer and fear had entered my relationship with your father big time. The main problem in my marriage was alcohol. Oh there had been other women as well, but alcohol was the constant theme and was your father's constant friend and companion. My stomach was constantly in a tight knot of apprehension as his behavior had become very predictably unpredictable and although I had been searching for some time, for a "cure" for his drinking problem, none was in sight.

You know, I really did have feelings for your father in the beginning. I am not sure now if it was love because I believe that true love never fades. I was happy when I got married and I believed that we would grow old together. When I married your dad, I felt like I was finally a part of a real family, a stay together family, and a close family. In some ways, it was almost like I married a family, at the very least I married into a family. Little did I fully realize when I separated from your father that I would lose this family and in some ways and for some years, you would also lose a big part of your family along with losing your dad.

Let's get down to the nitty-gritty. We actually separated on your fifth birthday, Daniel. Looking back, that was a really bad day to choose, but we did not choose it because it was your birthday, more because it was a Saturday. I was working full time and your dad was out of work. We both wanted to celebrate your birthday with you; your dad by this time was planning on going back down south to find work and had arranged with one of his sisters that he would live with her and her husband for a while. The weekend was the best time for him to move, as I was free to take you away from the house whilst he moved out. So on the Saturday morning, we took you on a farm visit for your birthday treat. It was the last time we would be together as a family for quite some time. Further down the track, we tried a birthday (your tenth, Sally) and a few Christmases, but they were mostly a disaster and we certainly did not turn out to be the happy separated family where mums and dads and stepmums and dads all get together and have a wonderful time!

You both loved looking at the animals and I seem to remember that you liked the café. Both of you were quite excited because we were due to go and visit my cousin Carol and her son, David. Carol is really more than a cousin to me; she has been more like a sister and best friend. It was her family I lived with when I first came to England and it was whilst living with her family that I became pregnant with my first child. When I was sent to London after the abortion, it was she that came to visit me and it was her that I eventually chose to confide in about what had happened. So it was that when she herself got pregnant as an unmarried teenager, she turned to me. I feel that I was able to tell her how awful having an abortion had been and to encourage her to keep her baby, which of course, turned out to be David. You both loved her as she is such fun to be with and you also looked up to her son, David, who being a little older than you, was very cool in your eyes. He always played with you both.

We planned to sleep there the night and return home in the morning. You knew that daddy was not coming with us and that he was moving out, but really you did not understand what this meant. Your dad and I separated at the end of the morning; I must have driven him back to the house where we had been living, which was now up for sale. I can't remember clearly the exact details of the day. I was just glad that he was finally going. You were of course, oblivious of the implications of what was about to happen in your family life. In a way, your world was about to turn upside down. Neither of you, nor me, fully realized the consequences of this decision. Life without a father would be very different from life with a father. In some ways, it would improve drastically, but in others it would cause devastating effects on you, Sally, as you have always felt abandoned by your father, but also on you, Daniel, as you have missed a father's firm guiding hand and good male example.

So why would I do such a thing? What led me to this decision?

I could no longer live with fear. I feared every day that I would come home and find that your father had been drinking again. I feared every day that I would come home and find that he was angry with me for something I had done or not done. I feared that if I was a few minutes late or the car broke down, I would have to endure hours of interrogation and accusations that I was having an affair. I feared every day that I would come home and find some part of the house or garden ripped up, knocked down or taken apart, so that we then had to buy the new carpet or do the renovation that your dad wanted, but which we could not afford. I feared that one day I would weaken and actually give up my job, refinance the house for a mad business scheme of his and end up with him twenty-four/seven with me doing all the work, caring for you both and with him ordering me about and drinking. I feared we would be homeless and bankrupt before long. I feared most of all that my children would grow up in a household of fear. I did not want that so I faced my fear of being alone and decided that that was better than continuing in my marriage.

I had loved being part of your dad's family. Your grandparents were wonderful people who really loved and cared for you both. They had accepted me into their family, shown me much kindness and for that I will always be grateful. In the end, however, as the saying goes, blood is thicker than water, so naturally they supported your dad and were upset with me. At first I tried to explain to them what it was like being married to your dad, and in their hearts they knew, but still, he was their son and they loved him and wanted us to get back together no matter what the marriage was like. There was no way I was going to expose my private humiliating life with their son to them, as they would not believe me. That is the way loyalties lay and in the same situation I would probably have felt the same as them.

So now you know it was more than the fact that your dad was an alcoholic; it was more than the fact that he had affairs. It was fear and a need for peace that drove me to separate from and finally divorce your dad.

All these years later, can you understand and forgive? I hope so because I love you and always wanted the best for you. Life was not turning out the way I planned it, but I thought we three would be okay.

All my love,

Mum

xxxx

LETTER 4

Life As a Single Mum

Dear Daniel and Sally,

Well, isn't it funny how sometimes what seem like the worst times turn out to be the best times. As I look back now on the years where it was just the three of us, I can see we had so many good times and were so close. As I sit now writing this letter, I am looking at some photos of the two of you; in one, you are both standing by one of the cars I had during that period, a red Nissan bluebird. It was an estate car with an electric sunroof and a large boot. I can't remember the exact occasion, but you are both standing at the side of the car. Although you are eighteen months apart in age, at this stage you could be mistaken for twins, not that you look alike.

Sally, you look wild and free, your stunning white blonde hair is being blown by the wind and your jacket is off your shoulders and hanging loosely by your elbows. You are dressed in jeans, T-shirt, and trainers. The trainers I know would have been yours from new as I did not believe in children wearing secondhand shoes. The clothes would all be from secondhand shops or be hand-me-downs from friends. Daniel, you look quizzical and faintly amused. Your thick blonde hair is short and neat with a heavy blunt fringe. You are wearing a thick bomber jacket with a collared T-shirt and thick fleece underneath, with tracksuit trousers and trainers. Your clothes, too, would have been hand-me-downs, although I may have bought your jacket because you were a lot fussier than Sally and very conscious of what you wore. You hated clothes from secondhand shops, but did not mind hand-me-downs from friends or cousins.

My guess is that you were about eight and nine in this photo. For some reason, I love it and it is one of the ones that I brought to Australia with me. Next to that picture and in the same frame is one taken a couple of years earlier. You both look so happy; a look of wild excitement is on your glowing face, Daniel, and Sally, you are giggling and bright eyed. I think this one was taken at the time of my parents' fortieth wedding anniversary, which was in October 1991. This would have only been about six months after your dad and I split up. We were in the small ex-council house in Bally Gardens that I bought on my own. It is the house that to me signifies most our times together as a threesome. Sally, you are wearing an OshKosh denim pinafore type dress with a

pink and blue check shirt underneath. I remember the dress for two reasons; you hardly ever wore a dress; and my sister bought it for you
from Canada when she came over to England for the Fortieth Wedding
Anniversary Party I threw for Nana and Granddad. She loved you both
to bits, but because you were a girl, Sally, and she had two boys, she
tended to satisfy her longing to buy little girl outfits by buying them for
you whenever we were able to see each other, which of course, was not
very often as she lived overseas.

You know that even though I was no longer with your dad, money
was still tight and apart from a period of about eighteen months, he
never paid any maintenance or contributed to your upkeep. I was working full time as a teacher and caring for you both. I loved the house in
Bally Gardens and it was just right for the three of us. Do you remember the wonderful neighbors that we had in the end house? They were a
married couple with three girls and I found out later that they were
Christians. About a year after we moved there, Sue came round to see
me and offered to have you guys before and after school if you moved
to the same school as her youngest daughter. She didn't want any
money for this, but in the end agreed to a token sum. She will never
know what a blessing this was for us as not only did it save me the
extortionate nursery fees I was paying, it also meant that in the morning
all I had to do was to take you next door before setting off for work and
all I had to do when coming home was pick you up from there. She
walked you to and from school and gave you afternoon tea before I
picked you up.

For those years, it was pretty much just the three of us all the time.
You both had to do all the same activities, as there was never anyone
else to leave you with. Apart from the working day, we were together
all the time. The things I remember the most were swimming, soccer,
and gym club. I have always loved swimming and when you could both
swim, there was nothing I loved more than taking you swimming. I had
to wait until you could both swim because my eyesight was so bad that
I could not see you in the pool without my glasses, and therefore could
not take you on my own before that time. (I had to give up wearing
contact lenses shortly after marrying your dad as I became allergic to
the contact lenses solution.)

We often used to spend weekends and holidays visiting my mum and
dad (Nana and Granddad), who had by then retired from active missionary work and were living in North Wales. These were the times I

loved because it gave me the opportunity to finally feel part of a family. It was at this time that I actually got to know my parents. Whilst visiting them, we would attend church with them, although at the time I had come to believe that God did not exist and that church rituals were an elaborate fantasy. I still felt that my father was a hypocrite for what had happened earlier in my life and I still felt a distance and coldness between us. He really just could not face talking to me about anything meaningful. He seemed to have sympathy for others in the same situation as me (single parents), but to me, he always said, "You made your bed; you lie on it."

Even though there was obvious enmity between us, I did feel that even if he didn't like me much and was ashamed of me in many ways, that in other ways he was proud and that underneath it all he loved me.

He was angry that I was not bringing you both up in a church setting and that I was not living a "Christian" life. He was upset that I utterly rejected everything that he stood for. Now, I realize that it must have been heartbreaking to him to know that I did not believe there even was a God. I remember saying to him, "We visit you often. Here is your opportunity to have some Christian input into your grandchildren's lives. When we are here, take them aside and tell them Bible stories and tell them tales from all your exploits in the jungle. Tell them what it was like when you first went out there and all the stories I have heard you tell other people about amazing events that happened. Tell them how you were rescued from the jaws of death on many occasions; tell them about being miraculously healed from cancer."

Somehow, he just could not do it. I came to realize that he just was not very good with children. He was a magnificent storyteller, but really only when center stage, teaching in front of an audience, in a pulpit or as the raconteur at a social gathering where all eyes and ears were on him. He could have told them the fabulous stories in a teaching situation, with them in a class and him at the front, but he could not do it in a personal situation either as father to daughter or as grandfather to grandchildren.

It was in these years that I got to know and love my mum. I saw the love that she gave both of you and although she was saddened by my failed marriage, she did not blame me for its end. She was the one who took time with you and took you outside to feed the birds with the scraps of food from the table, and to take apples to the horses in the field across the road from their little bungalow. It was she who made sure she bought the food you liked when we visited and it was she who came on all our little jaunts to the coffee shop in the town center, or the Pound shop on the high street. She came with us to the Nova swimming center, sometimes venturing in for a swim, sometimes just minding all the towels and bags whilst we swam. Just having that other adult there was so good.

It was Nana who came with us to Llandudno and walked down the pier with us and stood at all the puppet shows. It was she who came with us to the beach and sat on the sand making sand castles with you both. It was she who bought the buckets and spades ready there for when you visited and also bought balls that you could kick in her garden. I saw a side of my mum that I did not remember having when I was growing up. I guess retirement finally gives you the time to be a mum, which is why being a grandparent must be so sweet. (Plus of course, you can always give the kids back at the end of the day.)

Those memories are still sweet to me—are they sweet to you? Of course, the sweetest memories I have of those years when it was just us three are the two trips we made to Canada. They were truly magical. The first trip came about really because I had a car accident and suffered a whiplash. When the compensation money for the whiplash came through, I decided to spend it on plane tickets to Canada. I was so excited. I had visited there a few times during my college years when my sister was also in college and I had also visited there when my sister got married and been her bridesmaid, but had not been able to afford any holidays, never mind a trip to Canada, for many years. My sister and her husband had moved back to Canada after living and working as missionaries in Kenya. To you, they were Aunty Lina and Uncle Peter. They had two boys who were slightly older than you and were renting a house near the Bible College where Peter was now teaching.

On that holiday, your Uncle Peter taught you both how to ride bikes. A neighbor had a pool in their back yard and we spent many afternoons in their yard. This was in fact before you had learned to swim, Sally. Do you remember on the first visit we all piled round there and before I could even say "Jack Robinson," you ran to the pool, climbed on the diving board, ran to the end, and bounced into the pool. My heart was in my mouth, as I knew you could not swim. On the approach to the pool you had obviously seen the neighbors' boys jumping in and thought it looked fun. The look on your face as you surfaced after the jump was a sight to behold—total shock. By this time, I was at the side of the pool ready to jump in to help you to the side, but actually, you took a breath, moved your arms and legs, and made it to the side. Obviously, a natural swimmer! I pulled you out; boy, was I relieved. You didn't try that one again in a hurry and stayed in the shallow end of the pool for the rest of the swimming session. As for you, Daniel, I don't think I really spent much time with you that holiday. You and your cousins and their friends just spent the whole summer playing and having fun together, riding bikes, swimming, playing basketball, practicing catching baseballs, and playing with Fritz, the dog. We had outings to Niagara Falls, First Peoples reservations, shopping malls, Toronto, parks, churches, and you also went to a summer day camp with your cousins. On top of all this, we had a behind the scenes tour of the Africa encampment at Toronto Zoo where an old school friend from my Kenya days was now in charge. Sally, you did a lot of girly things with my sister and me, although I think most of the time you wanted to be with the boys. We all slept downstairs in the basement and had to contend with a few creepy crawlies, but apart from that, it was a great summer.

The second trip came two years later; we had enjoyed the first one so much that I put myself out to get the money for the second trip. By this time, your aunty and uncle had bought a house and were no longer living near the neighbors with a pool, but on this trip, we went up to Uncle Peter's family's cottage by a lake for a couple of weeks. There was no TV or shops, only a few board games and, of course, the natural countryside and lake to play in. What a time! No lifeguards in sight and open access to a lake. My heart was in my mouth for much of the two weeks as I was on constant alert for fear of someone drowning. Apart from that, it was idyllic. You guys spent most days in the lake sometimes swimming, sometimes boating (with us adults of course), and sometimes just jumping off the little jetty. There were frog-chasing outings and kitten-stroking sessions. We only had lake water so showers were a little murky, but who cared? These were the good times of our threesome life. I still look back on those holidays and regard them as some of the best of my life.

For the most part, I found single parenting very lonely, but I think that this was more because I did not have any close family back up. It was a relief to be able to make all decisions by myself and not to be hassled about where I went or what I did or what I chose in any given situation. I was in control, or so I thought. In reality, I was still very much not in control and my choices were in fact very limited, mostly by lack of finance, but I did have a real sense of freedom and a release from the fear that I had felt in my marriage. Being a lone parent is great in many ways: you can eat what you want, wear what you want, watch what you want, hear what you want, and allow or disallow what you want. There is no one to complain about anything that you do or do not do. On the other hand, there is no one to talk to about your children, his or her successes, slip-ups, triumphs, and tantrums. Especially being a teacher, I felt that I never talked to adults, always to children. There is no one else to get up in the night with a sick child, no one to be with the children when you have to attend parents' evenings either as a teacher or as a parent. There is no one to pop down to the shops to get that loaf of bread that you forgot to buy on the way home from work, so now it has to be a family outing.

I was realistic enough to know that if I had stayed married, I would also have basically been raising you as a single parent in that your dad probably would have continued to drink and so be an absent parent in another way. At the weekends, I would often get very lonely for adult company. When you are a single parent, friendships are hard to maintain. Other married people can be a little wary of you, as you are not in a "couple." Other single people without children are wary of you because you have children. You do not really have the freedoms of single life as you have the responsibility of children twenty-four/seven . In our situation, none of our close family lived near enough for me to drop in and visit. You had minimal contact with cousins or aunties and uncles as my sister lived in Canada and your father's family moved with him back down to London shortly after we split up. So, Daniel and Sally, I am sorry about that. I am sorry that in the split you did not just lose your dad living at home; you also lost the close proximity of your extended family.

In your preteen years, I remember happy times of celebrating birthdays at Pizza Hut. We made it our family tradition. I remember your friends James and Ali coming with us on trips to the swimming pool and also having sleepovers. You made friends at school and played with local children on the field at the front of the house. I hope that you can remember some of these times as happy times, as I do.

There was still a deep dissatisfaction in my life, a void, and also a feeling of human injustice. During the time we lived in Stoke, I worked as a Section XI teacher, which basically meant that I worked in mainstream secondary schools, teaching English as a Second Language. I got very involved with some of my students and their problems and also with their families. The majority of the pupils I worked with were originally from Kashmir (Pakistan) and I often got called "Paki lover." I felt a real empathy for these students making their way in a foreign culture and I felt much fulfilled in teaching them English. I could actually see that my teaching had an impact; no matter their intellectual ability, they all ended up being able to speak English, some better than others, but all could communicate on a basic level. This was still not enough for me; my job was always in jeopardy, in that the funding for our work was always in danger of being cut. On one occasion, I led a delegation to the Home Office to put a case for the continuation of the funding. At this time, I also got involved in Labor Party politics and in Teaching Union activities. I guess in a way, politics became my religion. I believed that I could help to change the world and make it a better place through these avenues.

I can really thank my parents for my belief that all people were of equal value. They were not political in any way, but the Bible had taught me that God loved all people and that all were worth saving. Although I did not share their faith in God, at that time, they had instilled in me the worth of all humanity. Their lives also showed a love of all peoples in that they dedicated their lives to helping the less fortunate, not only overseas in Africa, but also on their return. My father in particular was active in prison visiting and I found out after his death that he had spent much time visiting and preaching in prisons.

So, Daniel and Sally, my life at this time was really split into two compartments: work and home. At work, I became more confident and put a lot of energy into my job, I started to let myself become ambitious and started studying for a master's degree to further my chances of promotion. At home, I put all my energy into both of you. I found disciplining you hard and just kind of expected you to tow the line—my line—which of course, you did not, as you are only human. There was a constant rivalry between you both for my affection and time and I did my best to give to each of you equally. Now I live by a different premise and realize that fairness is not necessarily about treating people in exactly the same way; it is about giving each person what they need.

In some ways, I feel that I failed you both in that I did not give you that firm foundation and training that would have been best for you. Sure, I had rules; sure, I tried to make you obey them, but it was tough going. I was usually totally exhausted at the end of the day and emotionally drained. I had no down time as they call it nowadays. It really was all work and no play. Looking back, I feel the major problem I had was that I really did not know how to do the hard stuff. I did not know how to teach you gratitude and respect. Every instruction of mine that you did not like was a battle to enforce and I really did not have the parenting skills to be firm and fair. Looking back, it was just seemingly minor things, really, like getting you to come in from playing on time and you seemed to constantly fight with each other—I mean really fight physically. I could barely turn my back and you would be fighting. Of course, you always blamed each other for "starting it" and I never really knew who had. Sally, you always wanted to play with Daniel and his friends and in fact you often had the same friends. You loved the rough and tumble and enjoyed soccer and wrestling. I actually now realize that you were probably both stronger than me physically at quite an early age as I have come to recognize that I probably have low muscle tone and have particularly weak wrists. Physically, I felt completely drained all the time, but I carried on regardless.

The best time of the day for me was bedtime; you would both have a bath (you actually bathed together until you were about seven or eight) and then would put on your pajamas and come and lie on my bed with me. I would have you, Sally, on my left and you, Daniel, on my right. At first I read the same book to both of you, but as your tastes began to diverge, I would read part of a book that each of you had chosen. I loved that time; it was relaxing and warm, and I felt very close to you both at that time. From there you would go to your respective bedrooms and I would give you each some private "goodnight" time. Sally, you often asked me to pray with you and asked me why I did not believe in God. I would often end up praying even though I did not think my prayers were being heard, just to pacify you. Daniel, you always wanted me to stay with you until you were asleep and used to ask me to sing "Silent Night" to you, which I did most nights. These were indeed special times for me and I hope that they were for you, too. I hope I will never forget them.

At this time, my father was becoming frailer; he had a heart attack and also had prostate cancer. His osteoarthritis was becoming more incapacitating and he was having trouble driving his car, as it did not have power steering. An old injury in his left leg was playing up so that he could no longer feel anything below his knee. I was really worried that he and my mum would have a car accident, as he could not feel the clutch below his left foot. In 1995, I went to Chicago for eight days on a student exchange for the master's degree I was completing. It had been very difficult to arrange the trip, as I needed someone to look after you two whilst I was gone so I asked your father if he would look after you both for a week.

Your contact with your father had become spasmodic as he now lived in London. He had started attending AA and was allegedly sober and living with his parents, so I figured it was safe for you to visit during the holidays. I would drive down to London and drop you off and then drive straight back. I often did not even get offered a cup of tea when I dropped you off after a minimum of five hours driving. The visits always seemed to be at my instigation. I thought that it was important for you to continue to have contact with your father and was confident that being at your grandparents was a safe setting. I was, however, always made to feel that it was an inconvenience to them and that I was a bad person. I guess they were just sad that their son's marriage had not worked out. So when I needed to go to Chicago, I took the risk and asked your dad if he would come up to Stoke and look after you both whilst I was gone. He agreed to come up for part of the time and I was convinced that he was *dry* so that you would be safe. My parents agreed to take over from him for the last couple of days and to be there on my return.

When I came back from Chicago, I noticed that my dad was having trouble getting down the steps in our front garden to our front door and a week or so later I contracted someone to come and put a handrail in so that he could get down more easily. I also had a handrail put on the stairs inside the house so that he would also have something to hold onto if he needed to go upstairs when visiting. The trip to Chicago started to give me itchy feet; I looked into the possibility of going over there with both of you to work in the university whilst finishing my master's degree and doing a PhD. It was very tempting, but it turned out not to be possible because I was a single parent.

So as I said at the beginning of this letter, what seemed like the worst times from the outside actually have turned out to be some of the best times for us three. Although it was hard and very, very lonely, I loved you to bits. I held down a stressful full-time job as a secondary school teacher and even progressed in my career. I provided a roof over our heads and we always had food. Of course, we did not have the best clothes or latest car and most of the time we had quite an isolated life with not much going on socially for us as a family.

There were times when I felt that I could not go on and I felt aban-doned and alone in the world. These times were mostly on a Friday night after work. I would feel totally exhausted and would also long for adult company, or just to go out and have some fun. On these nights, I would sometimes sit on the floor in the kitchen smoking after the two of you had gone to bed. I occasionally had a bottle of wine and would sit smoking, drinking, and crying, wondering how my life had ended up the way it had. I guess I had a lot of underlying feelings of sadness and regret, which surfaced at these times. I wondered if my life would ever change.

The next morning, however, I would get up and get on with the day and kind of bounce back into life. You both kept me going at this time and I was determined to make you feel loved and wanted.

I hope that you both can look back on these days with some fondness and can remember the good times.

Love,

Mum

xxxx

LETTER 5

A Death in the Family/Moving to London

Dear Daniel and Sally,

The summer and autumn after I went to Chicago, three events took place that changed the course of all our lives forever. First, our next-door neighbors, not the ones who looked after you, but the ones on the other side of our house, went on holiday to Spain, and whilst they were there their oldest son was tragically killed by a freak wave whilst sunbathing on a ledge. It was really shocking as he was only eighteen, very good looking, well known, and popular in the area. I went to the funeral that was attended by about four hundred young people along with friends and family.

As if this was not enough to remind me of the fragile nature of life, one of my teaching friends died suddenly from lung cancer. She and I were not only friends at school, but had also started meeting out of school as you attended the same Gym Club as her children on a Saturday morning. We also started getting together socially, during holidays and weekends. We found we had a lot in common; besides being teachers, her children were similar ages to you two and her husband was a recovering alcoholic. She knew all about living with alcoholism and she was a smoker like me. (Even in those days, we were becoming a persecuted breed, forced to smoke in small dark rooms or outside and out of sight.) It is strange, but when I was a smoker, I always sought the company of other smokers. When it was banned from most workplaces and public buildings and you had to go to a designated smoking area, it promoted almost instant friendships with other smokers. The downside, obviously, was the extreme health risks and the hole in my finances. In my friend's case, no doubt it contributed to her early death. Oh and she was a Christian, which I was not, but I knew all about it, or so I thought.

She was involved in a minor car crash and suffered a whiplash injury and was off school for a couple of weeks. When she returned she told me that she had been having some chest pains, but her doctor had dismissed them as being symptoms of stress. Her chest pains continued and after a couple of months of returning to the doctor and being told not to worry, her husband took her for a second opinion. It was then that she discovered that she had terminal lung cancer, which they thought had been triggered by the car accident. Less than six weeks later, she was dead. Just before she died, she wrote a letter to all the staff at the school where we worked asking us not to be sad for her as she was a Christian and she was going to be with her Lord. I remember reading it and crying for her, for her husband, and for her children. I thought she was deluded. The funeral went by in a bit of a blur for me; I was really sad to have lost her and was very sad for her family. I wrote to her husband afterwards, but never saw him or the children again. He wrote and told me that people in his church were being very good and were helping him with the children.

The final blow of that year came on November 23 when my dad died whilst I was sitting with him in hospital. I was utterly devastated and the feeling took me completely by surprise. Two-and-a-half weeks earlier, he had been rushed into hospital with a blood hemorrhage and I had rushed over to Wales to be with my mum. He ended up having eight blood transfusions. For the next two weeks, I went to Wales daily whilst you were at school and neighbors and a couple of friends picked you up from school and looked after you until I returned home each night. My dad was in intensive care at first, but seemed to stabilize and was put in an ordinary ward. At the weekend, we all went down and stayed with my mum and visited Granddad in hospital. On the second weekend, he seemed to be recovering and was able to sit up in a wheelchair and speak lucidly. I remember you both talked to him for a little while and then went down to the day room to watch TV. It seemed as if he was going to make some kind of recovery. As we drove home later that night, I thought that the immediate crisis was over. I was worried about my parents' future as the doctors had been indicating that they were not sure my father would be able to continue driving and that he was going to need care twenty-four/seven for the foreseeable future. It all seemed very strange, as he had been up and running just a few weeks previously. My mother was considering how she would cope, but at that point we were mainly just relieved that he was making some sort of recovery.

Soon after I arrived home, but after you had gone to bed, my illusions were shattered. I received a distraught phone call from my mother who said that it had been discovered that my father had a blood clot in his leg, that it was very large, and that he was going to die, they just did not know when. He was now in a side ward by himself. My sister had already flown over from Canada and was staying with my mum. She immediately contacted her husband and started making arrangements for him and their boys to come over to Wales. I rang your dad and asked him to come up and look after you, which to give him credit, he agreed to do. The next day, I told you both the situation that your dad would be coming up to look after you and that I would be going down to spend time with Granddad in the hospital before he died. You both wanted to come with me, but I did not think it would be a good idea as my mum, my sister, and I would actually be staying at the hospital. I thought you would be bored and restless and I just wanted to spend time with my mum and sister and support them in their grief. At that time, I did not feel any grief. I was sort of on automatic pilot. I was sad for my mum, as I knew she would be devastated when my dad was gone and I was sad for my sister because I knew how close she felt to my dad even though they lived on different continents. I just felt numb inside and got on with the practicalities of making sure that you were cared for and that my work was aware of the situation. I wondered if my dad would be alert and awake when I arrived and also secretly hoped that he would say sorry to me for forcing me to have an abortion when I was eighteen. I really wanted him to respect me and not talk about me as if I was a worthless piece of scum. I always felt that he looked at me as if I was dirty and that I had completely failed his expectations of me.

I had not told you two about the abortion at that time, but your dad had told his family about it when we split up. Your grandparents on your dad's side were pro-life and he knew that telling them would make them think less of me. I had always found that to be hypocritical as your dad's oldest sister had also had an abortion, but none of the rest of the family knew and I sure wasn't going to be the one to tell them! Anyway, this was what was uppermost in my mind. I know that you especially, Daniel, have asked me since why I did not take you down to see your granddad again before he died. It really was because I thought it would be better for you if you remembered him as he was on that Sunday afternoon. I also just could not cope with the logistics of taking you both to the hospital and staying there. I thought I acted in your best interests though looking back, in this and other instances, I could have acted differently, but I didn't. You did not know about my past (the abortion) and I was hoping that my dad would realize that he needed to say sorry to me before he died. I did not want you to know about the abortion at that time.

The next few days were very tough for me. My mum and sister and I took turns to sit with my dad, who was by now very ill. We did round the clock, two-hour stints. He was no longer sitting, just lying on a bed floating in and out of consciousness. He must have been on very strong painkillers/medication. Previously when he had been in intensive care, he was not even speaking in English; he was speaking in Kiluba (an African tribal language) and French, two of the languages that he spoke fluently and that he had used extensively in his life for teaching and preaching. He was speaking in English now, but if I had been hoping for an apology, it was not to come. He was very weak and mostly he just requested water to drink. He did not complain and sometimes when I was with him, I sat and said nothing or read psalms from the Bible to him.

The day he died was a Friday and it was early in the morning. He suddenly took a very deep breath and his head rose off the pillow; he exhaled a long breath and it sounded strange, not like any other breathing I had ever heard and then he was gone. I immediately pressed the buzzer for the nurse to come and she confirmed that he was dead. I ran and woke my mum and sister and they came running to the room, crying. I went outside and chain-smoked. I felt completely numb and empty. So my dad was dead; what now?

What happened next took me completely by surprise. I had contemplated many times how I would feel if one or both of my parents died. As you know, Nana and Granddad spent most of their adult lives living in very dangerous situations. Firstly, they lived through World War II in England and endured bombing, blackouts, and rations. Then as missionaries in Central, Southern and Eastern Africa, they survived coups and civil wars at regular intervals. Two of their close missionary friends were martyred and others died as a result of disease including their very own first child (my sister). Even after their official retirement, they had returned to work in both Congo and Zambia and endured hardships and deprivations. On top of this, they had both had various health scares. So for this reason, I had thought about the possibility of their deaths many times. I had even contemplated my own death as I, too, had been at the wrong end of a gun. I did not think I would be too sad if my dad died because I felt as though he had abandoned me emotionally throughout my life. How would the lack of his physical presence on this earth be any different? How wrong can you be? I was totally and utterly struck down with grief over what could have been, indeed, what I felt should have been. He was dead and we could not restore the relationship. At the time, I could not even begin to describe how I felt. The way I coped initially was to try to be practical and help my mum to arrange a funeral. Everything seemed to be moving in slow motion, but at the same time speeding past. I almost had the same experience that I did when you were born, Daniel, except this time the feeling was not amazing joy. The world around me seemed surreal; everyone was just floating by and I was seeing it through a haze of intense grief. All that was going through my head was: *My dad is dead, my dad is dead, my dad is dead, my dad is dead, my dad is dead; don't you know my dad is dead!*

There was also intense relief that the grueling stay at the hospital was finally over. It was a Friday when he died and later that evening, I drove back home to pick you both up and bring you to Wales. Your own dad needed to get back to London and you wanted to be with me.

All during this time, I had been playing a Bob Marley tape in my car. Some of the songs I listened to were: "Don't Worry 'bout a Thing," "Three Little Birdies," "No Woman, No Cry," and "Exodus."

To this day, I am reminded of my dad whenever I hear any of those songs played, which is really weird because he would have hated Bob Marley's music if he had ever heard it. I no longer have the tape or the album, but may hear the songs randomly in shops or on TV and they make me want to cry.

These three deaths of my friend, our neighbors' son, and finally of my dad, produced a deep unsettling of my soul. I know that both of you were also affected by your granddad's death. Nana was given tranquillizers by the doctor as she was unable to rest or sleep and he also advised us that we should all look at my dad's dead body in the coffin, as it would help us all to bring closure to his life and accept his death. So following his advice and after my sister's two boys and her husband arrived from Canada, we all took a trip to the funeral parlor and had a look in the coffin. At the time, I truly believed it was the right thing to do, but I know that since then you, Daniel, have told me that it disturbed you deeply for years and you were angry with me for making you look because it became your last memory of your granddad. I am sorry about that. My intentions were good, but as is often the case, the outcome was not beneficial. Seeing my dad in the coffin did not have a bad effect on me. I knew it was only his body, but I had been with him when he died so the reality of his death was not an issue with me. I think for all of us that this was the time that the fragility of life struck home and we faced the fact, if only for a time, that death was a reality for all of us. Young people died, middle-aged people died and old people died; no one was exempt from the possibility. It certainly changed the way I approached life. I had been living "one day at a time" for many years and I continue to live that way even now, but I also reassessed my life and started to take a now or never approach.

Firstly, I had a lot of grieving and anger to get rid of, but I kind of repressed all my feelings at the time. I remember that there were a lot of people at the funeral and I remember arranging the funeral with my sister. It was held at the church that Nana and Granddad were attending at the time. I composed the Order of Service and wrote a short biographical memorial note on the back. My sister and Mum chose the music and organized the speeches, etc. You both got to spend time with your cousins that you would not normally have had. Lots of people were sending messages of sympathy to my mum and everyone was saying what a great man my dad had been. I did not see it that way.

How come everyone else thought he was so nice and yet he was nasty to me? How come he had time for every Tom, Dick, and Harry that crossed his path, but not for me, his daughter? How come he had gone and died on me without saying sorry? How come he had missed his prime opportunity to make amends and now it was too late? At the funeral, I could not stop crying; it was like a flood. Most people would have assumed that I was overcome with grief for the loss of my dad, but in fact, I was really grieving that I had lost him all those years earlier. I was grieving that now I would never gain his approval.

Of course, it is only now that I can more fully understand the emotions that I felt then. At the time, I just felt like a rug had been pulled from under my feet and I was attempting to stand on a very slippery floor. Your little brother now has a computer game called Mario Galaxy and he plays it on his Wii. I was watching him play last night and on one of the planets, there are mysterious dark holes that appear in the game and you have to make sure that Mario does not fall into one of these holes. You have to be very alert and game savvy to avoid falling and he was managing very well and learning from times when he did fall, but it made me think that that is what it was like for me after my dad died. All the known had become unknown and dark holes were appearing in unexpected places.

After the funeral, I returned home with you and went back to work. Life seemed very strange. I had been in the middle of completing my dissertation for the master's degree that I was studying for in my own time. I had sent off the first couple of chapters for approval and was all set to go to finish the rest. I remember getting back to the house and my first few chapters had been sent back with a few recommendations for improvement. Normally, I would have been excited at the feedback and it would have spurred me on to finish the work; instead, I shoved it in a filing cabinet without even properly reading it. About a year later and without ever looking at the months of research I had done, I threw the lot away; it just did not seem important any more. Perhaps my reason for the study was to somehow gain my dad's approval and now, of course, he was dead so it did not matter. I don't really know, but all I do know is that I no longer cared about the master's degree.

Your aunty, uncle and cousins stayed on with Nana until mid-December and we decided to celebrate Christmas before they left as we felt that you kids had had a pretty rough time of it all. We wanted there to be a positive memory of the trip and Christmastime has always been hard for our family as we rarely get to spend it together. So we got a tree, presents, and I cooked a traditional Christmas dinner. Nana came, but she was understandably out of it: still in a complete state of shock and not really realizing that Granddad was dead. Afterwards, we decided to go up to a well-known local folly on Mow Cop and explore and let you kids have a run around. Nana and your cousins were all going to drive back to Wales at the end of the outing and we were going to return home as they were due to fly back to Canada the next day.

This is probably a day that both of you remember and each of us will have different memories of the day because we are different people and each person sees things with a different perspective. For me it was an awful day and another day that was a catalyst for change in my life.

Even then, I was a bit of a helicopter parent and never used to let you two out of my sight, but on this day, I relaxed and allowed you both to run off with your cousins, as their parents were a little more relaxed about supervision. I was exhausted having prepared the Christmas dinner and everyone was sad, not only because of my father's death, but because our family was going to be apart again and my mum would now be alone in her home and would be facing the reality of my dad's death.

Of course, this was the one day to be vigilant and soon we heard screams. You had all gone into a restricted area that had steep falls and you, Daniel, had slipped down an escarpment. My heart was in my mouth and we all rushed to the scene. In those days, none of us had mobile phones, but we knew we needed to call an ambulance as you had fallen quite a distance and it was clear that you, Daniel, were injured because you could not move. Uncle Peter started to climb down to see if he could pick you up and Aunty Lina went to one of the nearby houses to see if she could ring an ambulance. The residents said that it would be much quicker if we took you to hospital ourselves as often the ambulances could not make it up to the top of Mow Cop and they had been known to get lost en route. Fortunately, Uncle Peter somehow managed to pick you up and climb up the side of the Cop. To this day, I don't really know how he managed this feat. You, Daniel, had blood all over one of your trouser legs and you were whimpering. Your face and arms were bruised and scratched and you had had a knock to the head in the fall. Everything was a blur and was happening so fast, yet again in slow motion; it is so strange what happens to our concept of time when we are in a crisis.

We managed to put you, Daniel, into the front seat of the car and Sally, you got in the back. I thought that everyone would come to the hospital with us, but as your aunty and uncle and cousins were flying the next morning, they had to go back to Wales. So we quickly said goodbye and I sped off to the hospital that was about twenty-five to thirty minutes away in Newcastle-under-Lyme. When we got there, I decided to go right to where the ambulances park as I knew that there was no way I was going to be able to go to the car park and carry you down. I did the right thing because as soon as I got you through the doors, a crash team was called and you were strapped to a stretcher with head restraints. No four-hour wait here—you were taken straight into the emergency section. You were immediately hooked up to drips to administer pain relief and provide fluids to your body. As I looked at you there all hooked up, recent memories of my dad dying came flooding back and I thought I was going to lose you. I started to go dizzy and faint. The staff revived me. They sat me down and gave me a drink of water. Then, Sally, you and I had to wait whilst the staff removed Daniel's clothes, gave him a full examination with x-rays and other tests. I vaguely remember that I went to get you, Sally, something to eat, but there were no hospital cafes open so I just got crisps and chocolate from a machine.

It was good news; the only real injury was a broken ankle and the rest was cuts and bruises. I was told that it had been a very lucky escape and that it was amazing that you, Daniel, had not suffered much more severe injury and indeed you had thwarted death by a fraction. Looking back now, I know that God had his hand on your life and that it was not your time to go. You were preserved for a reason.

We left the hospital late that night, with a pair of crutches and you, Daniel, with a lower leg and foot in plaster. It had been a clean break so no surgery was needed. You had been given morphine for the pain whilst in hospital, but this began to wear off and you were in a lot of pain for the next few days.

I was totally emotionally exhausted after losing my dad and then nearly losing you. I wondered how I would cope with looking after you and continuing to work as by this time, I had had quite a bit of time off with my dad's death. I ended up taking you to work with me for a few days before the schools broke up for the Christmas break. At this time, I decided that I could no longer cope alone and that something would have to change. I started to think about moving back to London as your dad and his family had moved back there. I was fed up with my job as I had moved from being a Section XI teacher to working for the school on staff as a Special Needs teacher. Although being promised English work, I found I was teaching a lot of special needs mathematics and I felt incompetent in this area. Promotions had been promised, but had not materialized and all the freedoms that went along with my previous responsibilities had vanished. It was time for a change.

It is true that hindsight gives us a different perspective on events. Looking back, I can see that moving to London was traumatizing for the two of you. I personally thought it would be good for you to be able to see your dad, whom I had been told was now sober and going to AA. I also felt that it would be great for you to feel connected to his family, as our family was now just Nana and us. It was almost as if my dad's death had lifted all restraints from me. I started applying for jobs in London and got one on my second interview. An old friend of mine from my days of teaching in Brixton was a teacher there so I was quite happy, although I realized that it was a very rough boy's school. We were going to be able to live near to where I used to live. Before we moved, my personal life became crazy. I started living a double life. I truly drowned my sorrows on a few occasions and started going to nightclubs and dated a few men I met there. They were all highly unsuitable, mostly younger than I and only really after sex. It is a time I am very ashamed of, my wild time if you like. It was like I was making a statement: Okay life sucks, everyone treats everyone else like dirt, so I am going to give as good as I get. I could die tomorrow so why not party at every available opportunity? I was sick of staying in and being "good." So when I got the opportunity, I went out and sometimes stayed out. Of course, I only did this if I had managed to get you baby-sat or you yourselves were having a sleepover somewhere, or if you had gone down to London to be with your paternal grandparents.

I was never going to earn my father's approval now; he was dead, so why not just be the person he obviously thought I was? I became very rebellious inside. Why should I stick around in Stoke? I had only moved there because your dad had wanted to move out of London to study and my mum and dad had a house there that they needed someone to rent. Then when my mum and dad came back to live in their house and I needed them to be close for once in my life because of all the problems I was having in my marriage, they moved away even though I begged them to stay around! I had been a smoker since I was eighteen and had given up a few times, but at this point, I started to smoke heavily and I also started to lose weight. It seemed to be just falling off me. I went to the doctor because I started to get a little concerned and she told me that I ought to be grateful as so many women try to lose weight. Why should I be concerned if I was managing it without even trying?

You both seemed to be quite excited about moving and I found a school and a child minder for you before we moved. I put the house on the market and hoped for the best. The house didn't sell as the market was on a downturn so I decided to rent it out. I felt a little guilty about moving so far away from my mum, but I offered for her to come with us and she declined so that assuaged my guilt. There were a few worrying signs that I should have noted, but I thought moving would solve my parenting problems. Daniel, you had already been in trouble with the police and you were becoming very hard for me to handle. You always resisted authority, whether it was teachers, police, or mine. You just did not accept no for an answer and seemed to have no reverence for anyone. You had no fear of consequences. However, you had another side, a scared side. After your accident, you started sleeping in my room on a mattress on the floor and when we moved to London, this continued. I used to find at night after I had put you to bed that you would sneak downstairs and sit just outside the living room door on the floor. You did not like to be upstairs if I was downstairs or downstairs if I was upstairs. The belligerent daytime boy was quite different after dark.

Sally, you adored your brother and always wanted to be with him and his friends, even at school. You seemed to be very happy-go-lucky and had a certain confidence about you. I can remember sending you to your room as a punishment and up you would go quite happily. You wouldn't even want to come out when the time out was over, which I found quite frustrating. Both of you nagged me to death about my smoking. I didn't smoke in the house until you had gone to bed, but I did smoke in the car or when we were out and you were both constantly pretending to choke and open all the windows and give me lectures about the evils of smoking. This, of course, completely blinded me to the fact that you both started smoking yourselves very young. Even now, I do not know when you started because I have only found out recently some of the things that you got up to whilst growing up.

Before we moved to London, we cleared out the house and did a car boot sale of all the toys and games that you no longer played with. We only made thirty-five pounds, but I let you split the money between you. We left minimal furniture in the house for rental purposes; friends helped us load a minivan with some personal possessions and off we went on our London adventure. All of this had been prompted by the three deaths, particularly my dad's and had culminated in your accident, Daniel. I was seeking satisfaction and never finding it. I was seeing a futility in life and wanting to fill a void before it was too late. I thought that career satisfaction and having fun would do the trick. This is what I hoped to achieve in London. Blindly, I thought that you both having more contact with your dad, who was allegedly a reformed character, would take the pressure off me and also give you both the opportunity to have that relationship with your dad that I had lost with mine. It all seemed so important then. I really wanted you to have something valuable so that you would not end up like me inside. My father's death taught me how valuable fathers are and how much they can influence their children. Children need mothers and fathers. I believe that there is a reason that we come from male and female: boys and girls need both male and female input into their lives. Now that my dad was dead, it seemed there was no male input into your lives and I felt that you needed more contact with your father and grandfather.

Daniel, you in particular in more recent years have lambasted me for moving, firstly down to London and then for moving back to Stoke after my second marriage. I hope this letter somehow explains my reasoning for the move; it was with good intentions and I always thought it would benefit you both. I particularly thought that it would be good for you, Sally. You and your dad had not had the best of relationships, partially due to the circumstances surrounding my pregnancy and your birth. This, I believed, would be the time when you and your dad could bond as father and daughter. I was so naïve; forgive me. I wanted something for you that I did not have myself and was grieving over now that my own dad was gone.

We make lots of decisions as parents that influence our children and others always tell us: your kids will be fine, they are resilient, and they are tough. Whereas I do believe that this is true, I now know that more preparation for the move would have benefitted all of us. Most changes can be coped with if we are well prepared and supported through any grieving or loss that we feel. Although the move to London proved to be more traumatic than I could have imagined, I believe that some good came out of it and now that I am a Christian, I know that God had his hand on us all the time.

All my love,

Mum

xxxx

LETTER 6

Dating Again

Dear Daniel and Sally,

Moving to London was not all that I expected it to be. My new job was very challenging. I was Head of Department in a large state boy's school in London. Many of the boys there were behaviorally challenged to say the least. The way I describe it nowadays is National Front skinhead, meets Somali refugee. Both groups of young men were mostly from highly disadvantaged families and were angry at life, the establishment, in fact anything representing authority (including school) and each other, but for different reasons. Many of the Somali refugees had seen close family members brutally murdered by machete and had left home and everything they knew and held dear to live in London. Many of the white youth came from homes and areas of high unemployment and had been fed the rhetoric from an early age that any ills they suffered were the fault of immigrants, who had taken all the good homes and jobs away from them, the rightful owners. The fact that many of the white boys were in fact also children of immigrants who had fled Europe under Hitler seemed to escape them as they associated the word *immigrant* with dark-skinned people. So classroom management was tricky, especially for a white woman in a very male environment. There were only a few women teachers and we had to prove our worth not only in the classroom, but also in the staffroom. My subordinate was a young guy who was in fact a very good teacher, but he was very unhappy that I got the job over him and never really supported me in the way he should have. That was the downside.

On the upside, I met up with a few teachers that had worked in the same school as me in Brixton when I had first started teaching and was able to reconnect with them. Probably because the school was such a challenging environment, once you got over the chauvinistic attitudes of some of the staff, they were all very friendly and organized lots of social events (think drinking sessions). I was, however, beginning to feel that I was ready to start dating again. I felt as though life was passing me by and that I would wake up one day at age fifty and discover that I was single and that both my children had moved on and were living their own lives. A few years after your dad and I separated, we got divorced and so I felt I was free to meet other people. The move to

London had not dissipated my feelings of dissatisfaction, and yes, you were now seeing more of your dad and your other relatives, but still I felt really alone. I was not really part of any family group although now at least you had grandparents and cousins and had started to regularly sleep over at your dad's.

He rose to the occasion of you coming to London and got his own flat where you both could stay. Every other weekend, you stayed with him and also every other Wednesday night. For the first year we lived in London, I believe he really tried to be the dad he should have been all the time. He even paid the out of school hours child-minding fees that had to be paid in order for me to go to work. We made an agreement that he would pay the child-minder directly. I was very pleased with this arrangement. For the first time since I met him, he was actually contributing financially to the upkeep of his children. I started taking you to soccer club on a Saturday and he also got involved in this and even started taking you himself and started to do some coaching. I believed him when he told me that he was no longer drinking and therefore allowed you both to spend time with him.

Of course, subsequently, you have both told me that he had not in fact given up drinking, but that he put you both under pressure not to tell me that he was still drinking. So you dutifully kept your mouths shut and did not let his secret out. I don't blame you for that; most kids would have done the same thing. On one occasion, he wrote me a letter asking if there was a chance of us getting back together again after I invited him for Christmas dinner. I realized that he had mistaken my civility and my attempts at being friendly and polite for your sakes as meaning that I was being friendly because I liked him. This was not the case. I found every encounter with him very awkward because I had truly lost all feelings toward him as a result of him totally humiliating me, emotionally, verbally, physically, and sexually throughout our marriage. I could never trust him again due to his unfaithfulness, but also due to his deceit and lies. I did, however, feel that he would and could be a better dad than he was a husband and that you deserved to know that side of him. I still don't know if I was right or wrong to pursue him to get to know his children, but what is done is done. In the meantime, every other weekend I was free to go out if I so desired.

At first, I just went out drinking with other staff members from work, but I found this very unsatisfactory, and all I ended up with was an occasional hangover. There was no one at work with whom I could envisage having a relationship. I did not want to meet up with men who were out drinking looking for sex so I decided to join Dateline.

It was quite exciting. I received a list of men with whom I was supposed to be compatible and I contacted them first by phone or letter. In return, others contacted me, either by phone or letter. There were no pictures, just a list. Some sent photos, most didn't, so I just had to judge whether or not to arrange to meet them by the sound of their voice. I did not have Internet connection—no Skype or Facebook; I did not even have a mobile phone. Hard to imagine nowadays, I know, but nothing was *instant;* everything took time. Communications were by landline phone or snail mail. Sometimes, it would be a few weeks before I would answer a letter or indeed receive an answer from someone. I confided in a colleague at school that I had joined Dateline and every time I arranged to meet someone, I gave her the person's details and told her where and when we were due to meet. At the end of the date, I would ring her to let her know I was home and if I didn't ring she was to call the police. I was very suspicious of any man that wanted to date a single mother and never introduced any of the people I met briefly to you. Of course, you do know one of the people I met at this time because it was Leroy.

So, yes, I have lied to you about how Leroy and I met. I feel really guilty about this. I remember telling you both that I had joined Dateline and that I was feeling lonely and wanted to meet other people to go out with. In fact over the years, you had both encouraged me to go out with other men. I remember one day in particular (before we moved to London) when you were about six and seven years old, both of you had been keen for me to have another baby because you wanted a little brother or sister. I had told you that I couldn't have a baby on my own; it took a man and a woman to make a baby. This satisfied you until one of your friends at school's mum got pregnant and married her boyfriend. The friend had a new baby on the way and a new daddy to boot. You were both so excited; you came rushing to meet me when I picked you up from after-school care and told me that we could have another baby, because I could marry someone else. It was like you had both had a moment of enlightenment: want another baby—get Mum to meet another man, they can get married, have a baby and we can have a new daddy. Hey, presto, all our problems solved. Yippee. Sorted! If only life were that simple.

So, I like to think that I was an honest parent who didn't hide things, but looking back, I can see that I was not honest about this. You knew that I had joined Dateline. You knew that I had had a few dates, but that I did not like any of the people I met. You knew that I had also met someone from Stoke who had come down to see me. When I met Leroy and basically fell in love, I somehow did not want you to know that I had met him through Dateline because I was embarrassed that you would naturally tell other people and that they would look down on me and on you guys. It is not such a big deal nowadays as so many people get involved with Internet dating, but then it was a big thing. So because I was embarrassed, I told you that I had met Leroy at a station in London whilst waiting for another date from Dateline who did not show up. It somehow seemed more romantic, a bit like falling in love at first sight. I did meet him at a station, but he was the date I was waiting for. Before I met him, we had been writing to each other and I had spoken to him quite a few times on the phone, so we had been in contact for a couple of months before we actually met. I am sorry that I lied about this, and I hope that you will forgive me. Maybe you knew already because I know that Leroy told Leo (Leroy's son from his first marriage) and Leo in turn may have told you. He never wanted to keep the way we met a secret; it was I. Recently, I have told a few people the truth about how we met and I am glad it is now out in the open. It is no big deal; lots of people meet in lots of different ways and no way is particularly right or wrong.

The day we actually met was quite amazing. We actually met at a London Railway station. I was instantly attracted to Leroy; he had lovely sparkly eyes and a lovely smile and had short-gelled hair. I had already fallen in love with his Scottish accent over the phone. My main concern was that I had not told him that I was a smoker and I knew that this would have to come out sooner or later. I knew that for some people this would be a big turn off, but I was not prepared to pretend that I did not smoke even if I did really like Leroy. As Leroy did not know the area very well, I had to decide where we should go first and even though I am not a fan of pubs, it was the only place I could think of where we could just have a quiet chat and see how we got along in person. The first thing that amazed and impressed me was that Leroy ordered a sparkling water to drink and bought me a lager, which I had requested. In my head I was thinking: *How refreshing—a man who drinks water in a pub.* It immediately put me at my ease and allayed any fears that I might have about him being a big drinker.

I had been told by many people that because I had already been married to an alcoholic, that I was over sensitive to other people drinking and considered them to be alcoholics if they had more than two drinks. I myself had given up drinking altogether during the last few years that I had been with your dad as I considered that alcohol had brought so much despair and unhappiness to our lives that it was best to just stay away from it completely. However, after my dad died, I had started drinking again socially and had even drunk to excess on a few occasions. Can't say it ever did anything for me apart from making me feel ill the next day when I still had to face life the way it was before I got drunk, but I guess it helped me to forget for a while.

The first few weeks were amazing. Leroy continued for the first few dates to only drink water. Then he started to drink, but not every time we went out. He never seemed to get drunk and seemed to be very sensible about his drinking. If he had had a few drinks, he always finished off the evening with drinking a couple of pints of water. I was not really worried. Here was someone who romanced me, sent me flowers, and bought me chocolates. He wrote me letters and phoned me often. We would talk for hours on the phone and when we met, the time melted away. He always seemed so positive and hopeful about life and was constantly thinking of places we could go and things we could do together, not only as a couple, but also with you. So he did drink a little and was not the teetotaler I had imagined when we first met, but he seemed to be very sensible with his drinking and he never appeared to be drunk. I was not unduly concerned. He was so intense and paid me so much attention, I was completely bowled over. He also had a boy of his own who was the same age as you, Daniel, and I noticed that he was a very loving dad. He regularly contacted his son and also paid maintenance to Leo's mum. As far as you two were concerned, he seemed to be kind and thoughtful. He was always trying to think of places to take you on the weekends that you were not at your dad's. You both seemed to get on with him quite well.

Not long after we met, Leroy started talking about getting married. I have to tell you both that this was not my intention when I joined Dateline. I actually just wanted to go out with someone who treated me well and took me out to dinner, theater, etc. I was not looking for someone to marry and I certainly was not looking to have more children. However, something changed when I met Leroy. I felt that he was a man that I could trust. He treated me very respectfully and seemed to accept me just as I was. I can't really explain it except to say that he made me feel like I had never felt before in my life. I felt sexy and beautiful. I liked the way that he did not interfere with the way I was bringing you two up and did not criticize me at all. In fact, as the relationship progressed, he often said, "You look after your children and I will look after you." He told me that he did not want to confront either of you, as the last thing that he wanted was to replace your dad. It was clear from the beginning that he was looking for a long-term relationship and that he wanted more children, but I did not expect things to move as fast as they did.

They say that love is blind and looking back, I should have seen the signs that alcohol was a problem for Leroy, but in my defense, I was not with him all the time and only saw what he drank when he was with me. I now know that he was a binge drinker, but at the time it just seemed to me that sometimes he drank and sometimes he didn't, so that indicated to me that he did not have a problem. The only experience I had had with alcoholism was with your dad and he was an everyday drinker. It was rare for him to go a day without drinking, but Leroy went weeks at a time. I did not realize that planning for the next drink motivated even the non-drinking times. I did notice that when he drank on a Friday, it usually continued on the Saturday and the Sunday, but quite honestly, I had a lot of friends at the time that did the same thing. In fact, a lot of the teachers I associated with not only drank at the weekends, but also smoked dope. One of my closest friends at the time also used speed to give her a pick up after drinking and using dope at the weekends, so that she could face her classes on the Monday. I myself at various times had had the occasional joint, mostly given to me by other teachers after going out for drinks on a Friday after work. So I really only thought that Leroy was drinking like many of the people I knew and hung out with at the time. I was a single parent, living and working in a tough state boy's school in London, and it was a hard job. I found it extremely stressful and just wanted to unwind at the weekends and I assumed it was the same for everyone else.

The move to London had not been an easy one for the two of you or even for me. Both of you had been quite stressed by the move and I had not expected this as I thought that being near your dad and your other relatives (grandparents, cousins, etc.) would compensate for moving schools and home. Daniel, you were becoming very hard for me to manage for a number of reasons. You wanted to go back to Stoke and on a few occasions actually slipped out of the house and started walking down the road saying that you were going back to Stoke. In the back of my mind, I was always worried that you would run away and was constantly checking on your whereabouts if you went out to play. I never allowed you out of the front of the house without my supervision and our back garden was not very big. The streets of London were not very safe and the neighbors were not friendly. The layout of the house we rented was not working for us, as there were two bedrooms upstairs and one bedroom downstairs. As the oldest, I wanted you to sleep downstairs, but you were too scared, so initially I put you and Sally in the same bedroom, but that did not work as you argued too much. It ended up that I put all your stuff in the bedroom downstairs, but you actually slept in my bedroom on a mattress on the floor. You had a real fear of the dark and of being alone and in the evenings, you would not stay in bed until I went to bed. It was like you had two personas: in the day you were over-confident and pushing the boundaries, but at night you were a softy, just wanting to be with mum. Sally also was having problems to the extent that I could not even go to the toilet or have a bath when either of you was awake in the house without her banging constantly on the bathroom door asking to be let in.

I don't know what name you would give her anxiety or yours. Obviously, you both were traumatized by the events in your lives, but could not actually verbalise them and rationalize why you were feeling the way you were. Perhaps your dad leaving had made you fearful that I would leave. Perhaps the three deaths of people that you knew made you realize that death comes to all of us and that you don't have to be old to die. I don't really know, but I knew that I was struggling to cope on my own in all ways, emotionally, physically, and financially. I have respect for every *single parent* out there, especially women who form the majority of single parents and whom society does not treat as well as single parents who are men, who are often regarded as heroes. In fact, they are all heroes; raising children is the job with the highest responsibility on the planet, has the longest hours, and is not paid.

I was actually also very lonely and still coming to terms with my dad's death. Leroy seemed to provide all the solutions to my life, I loved him, he loved me, and both of us believed in marriage and did not want to just live together. I thought that it would provide stability to both of you to be in a two-parent family. Everyone around me counseled me that if I was happy then it would rub off on the two of you. I didn't really do any research into stepfamilies or think very deeply about any of the pitfalls. I do remember talking to you both about getting remarried and neither of you seemed to object or have any strong feelings either way. You both said you liked Leroy and you really had no reason to dislike him at that time. He never interfered in your upbringing; in fact, life got better because he bought you treats much more frequently than I ever did. He also organized days out to theme parks and day trips to France. It all seemed so right.

Love,

Mum

xxxx

LETTER 7

Oh No! Another Alcoholic! — The Truth Hits

Dear Daniel and Sally,

What can I say? I divorced your father due to his alcoholism, and then married another alcoholic seven years later. You have a very naïve mother, to say the least. The first year of my marriage to Leroy was his final year of drinking, which was in fact his worst year of drinking. Lucky us! So now we were dealing with not just one alcoholic (your dad), but also two (your new stepdad)!

It actually did not take me that long after the wedding to figure out that Leroy had a huge problem with alcohol. We married in November 1997 and by New Year's Eve of the same year, I knew. There were a few occasions before we married that he drank excessively, but I put that down to various incidents that preceded the drinking, i.e., stress after a car accident, fear of flying on our return from a holiday in Greece, etc. It is not just alcoholics that are full of excuses for their drinking; it is also sometimes their spouses or families and I was no exception. I consoled myself with the fact that Leroy did not drink every day, and that he was not aggressive when drunk. Here was an alcoholic who *controlled* his drinking. Ha, ha, what a joke! Anyone who knows anything about alcoholism knows that it is drinking that controls the alcoholic and not vice versa, but I continued in my delusion.

Just prior to our wedding, Leroy quit his job and was still looking for another one when we got married. It was not long before he found work and he got a very good job working in Central London. It was amazing that he got the job because, if I remember rightly, he went to the interview as drunk as a skunk. That was the thing about Leroy: when he was drinking, on the whole he did not appear to be drunk. He did not slur his words or stagger and was not aggressive. He just consumed enormous amounts of alcohol and it seemed as if he would never stop drinking. He just removed himself from life, distanced himself from me, and drank. At these times, he did not really want to be with anyone and would just sit in the bedroom drinking, often listening to the same musical track over and over again.

So really what it meant for you two was that we continued life as before. I was still a single parent and you did not really have a stepdad;

it was more like he was mum's husband to you. He didn't really interfere with your lives apart from to buy you sweets or gifts. On the weekends that he was not drinking, he continued to arrange trips to the coast
or to a theme park or even day trips to Calais in France. I had a lot of
money worries at the time as I had not sold the house in Stoke and was
renting it out, but my main concern was the fact that I realized that
Leroy was an alcoholic. I started ringing my old contacts from Al Anon
who gave me support and counsel. I did not tell any of my friends or
family what I thought, as I felt like a complete and utter idiot. This did
not detract from the fact that I loved Leroy; I just thought I had made
yet another horrendous decision that was going to bring more disaster
to my life. Ever since I married your own dad, I had been living one
day at a time and I continued to do this. Somehow life is more manage-
able if you just have to cope with the one day you are living.

Looking back, I recognize now that Leroy saved most of his binges
to the times when you two were at your dad's. I do not know if this was
intentional, but I do remember that most times when I thought that he
and I would have some quality time alone together without me having
to be at work that it ended in disaster with him just drinking. One of
these times was the New Year after we married. Leroy had managed to
secure a really good job and was working in the City of London, which
was only really a short commute from where we were living. We had a
quiet Christmas day with just the four of us and Leo did not come down
from Scotland as he had only recently been for a visit. Leroy was not
drinking and the night before, because you two could not sleep, he suggested just after midnight that we allow you to open a few of your presents so that you would then go to sleep. (He was always having crazy
ideas like that and it made him fun to be with.) You could not believe
your luck, opened some presents and were then so tired that you both
slept in on Christmas morning.

You were due to spend New Year with your dad and his side of the
family and Leroy and I were going to take the opportunity to go back
up to Stoke-on-Trent. The second lot of tenants in my house had not
been paying the rent and I had informed them I was coming up to collect some money from them personally. I was looking forward to the
trip and both of you were looking forward to spending some time with
your grandparents and other relatives. But—and it is a big but—on
Boxing Day whilst the four of us were out in Bromley, purportedly to
look at the Sales, as we were about to pass the first pub on the high
street, Leroy said that he was going in for a drink and that he would see

us all later. My heart sank, as this had not been part of my plan for the day. This was about the time that I began to realize that booze was a real problem for him. I now realized that he was not going to have *a drink,* but I still hoped that it would only be one session. My hopes were not realized as that drink was the start of an almighty binge. The following day, your dad came and picked you up and after you had gone I started to get ready to drive to Stoke. I was still hoping that Leroy would stop drinking and come along as planned but he urged me to go without him, so I did. I told him that I would be back on New Year's Eve, as I wanted to spend it with him.

Over the next couple of days, I made excuses for his absence by saying that he was not very well. I did not get any money from the tenants. They offered me checks, but as the chap had "left his check guarantee card in his desk at work," I knew that they were not worth the paper they were written on. This later proved to be true as they all bounced. My heart was filled with trepidation, but I was anxious to return to London to see Leroy. I had spoken with him on the phone and he said that he had stopped drinking and was looking forward to my return. When I got back to the flat, I realized that this was not the case. Our bedroom floor was literally covered with beer cans, most empty, but some had liquid in them. (Turned out the liquid was in fact where Leroy had peed into the cans, as he could not be bothered to leave his drinking den and go to the toilet.) Leroy was not welcoming to me and basically told me to go out and enjoy New Year's Eve without him, as he was busy.

I went out with a friend from school and I must admit I had a few drinks myself that night. I had been married six weeks and what a mess it was. So you see, kids, I am not as clever as you might imagine; I had got myself into another almighty mess. What was I to do? Should I cut and run? Should I show myself up for the idiot that I was or should I hang in there and believe that this time it would be different?

Of course, the next day, Leroy started to come down off his bender and was very loving and apologetic. He admitted that he had a problem with alcohol and said that he would try to stop drinking. He devised a plan that we should keep all our weekends very busy, as the reason he drank was that he had nothing else to do and was bored. My fears started to subside and I thought that there was hope after all. I now know that that New Year's Eve was an absolute nightmare for him. Not only had he been mugged at a cash point whilst getting out money for some more booze, but he also was so far into the booze that he had visions of demons coming out of the walls of our flat. He had been well and truly frightened by what his drinking was doing to his mind and also to his physical well-being.

I have discovered that what a drinker will tell you often bears no resemblance to what they are actually experiencing or thinking. They live a life of lies, deceit, and cover up, and whoever lives with them has to be careful that they do not follow suit. Of course, I was already lying by not telling the truth about Leroy being sick. I was putting on a brave face to the world, whilst inside I was shrinking with despair and fear. I was kind of living a double life. On the outside, I was continuing as normal, looking after you two, going to work, pretending that everything was good; on the inside, I was a mess. My pride had pre-eminence. I was not going to admit the mess I was in to anyone. (I was hardly admitting it even to myself.) You see, when Leroy was not drinking, everything seemed okay and I put his drinking problem out of my mind.

The two of you were now in separate schools for the first time.

Daniel, you were in your first year of high school when I married Leroy. It was not the local secondary school, but I had appealed and got you into the nearest secondary school that had the best reputation. A teacher friend of mine had a son that was attending there and she recommended it to me. You seemed to be getting on quite well, but there were soon signs that your progression through high school was not going to be smooth when you were suspended for a day before the first term completed. Fortunately, I found the letter in your bag, as you had not intended to let me know you were suspended; instead, you told me, you were just going to pretend to go to school and hang around the streets until it was time to go home. I was horrified at the thought of you being on the streets, but it didn't seem to worry you at all. At the time, I would not even let you go out of our front door on your own without adult supervision, never mind wander the streets! When I asked you what you had been suspended for you told me that you had said something rude about the teacher under your breath and when they asked you to repeat it, you did—very loudly—and as it was rude and you would not back down, you were suspended. As a teacher, I knew that this was a bad sign as Year Seven pupils usually had more respect for teachers than you were showing. Of course, I still had to go to work so you had to come to school with me and sit in my classroom whilst I taught. The next day, a few of the boys were asking me about the "feisty kid" who sat in my classroom. So although a few alarm bells were ringing regarding school, you seemed reasonably happy to me, had friends and a keen interest in playing football.

Sally, you were still in primary school and seemed to have a lot of friends. You joined the African club at school much to the amazement of the other children in the club (all of whom were black). You insisted that you had a right to be there because your mum was born in Africa so that made you by default—African. I guess you had a point and they accepted you in the club. At this time, you and Leroy seemed to get on very well. You even sent us little notes commemorating our love. Your bedroom in the flat was tiny, but you never complained. Leroy bought you a second-hand TV, which meant that we now had two TVs which meant that there was no longer any need for Daniel and you to argue about what you wanted to watch. I don't actually remember there being a lot of arguing between the two of you at this time. Whether this was because I was so taken up with Leroy or whether it was just that you were getting along fine, I don't know.

Sally, I do remember that you were not keen on visiting your dad. You often asked if you could remain at home, but I made you go. I was still on the quest of trying to cement a relationship between the two of you. The lowest point in the relationship had been the previous year on your ninth birthday, before I had even met Leroy. You had asked that we all go out together—your dad, Daniel, you and me—to Pizza Hut in Bromley. I left the three of you at the table whilst I went to get some menus and when I returned your dad was shouting and you were crying. There had been a disagreement between you and Daniel and your dad had punched you. I was horrified and we all left the restaurant. We ended up going somewhere else, but all I wanted to do was scream at your dad and go home. I desperately tried to keep calm so as not to completely ruin your birthday, but looking back, I probably should have screamed at him as your birthday was already ruined. Daniel and he seemed to get on well, but there was still a barrier, it seemed, between the two of you. I believed that the incident on your birthday was isolated and you have never told me otherwise, because if I had even suspected that he was physically abusive to you, I would never have allowed either of you to see him. I know now that he was continuing to drink, but at the time I believed his lies and I also expected his family to tell me if he was drinking because they knew that the condition of him having access to you was that he was sober. Daniel and you have both told me that he continued to drink, but told you not to tell me because it would mean that he could not see you. This was partly true, but not entirely, as all it would have meant was that you were back to supervised access and that he could only see you if either your grandparents of one of your aunties was also there.

Of course, you were no angel—I remember finding some obscene graffiti in our bathroom written in ballpoint pen. It matched graffiti I had seen on some lampposts in our street with Daniel's name on it, so of course, he got the blame and a punishment. No matter how hotly he denied it, I did not believe him. Turns out you were the culprit, but I did not find out until much later on.

When we first moved to London, I had enrolled you both in a soccer club on a Saturday. For the first year, I took you along, but your dad was now getting involved and he was taking you both along. I believe he also started to coach one of the teams. He had bought a one-bedroom flat in Sydenham, which he was doing up and for a while, you were both going there every other weekend. It seemed to be working out well. When you were with your dad, you were also spending time with your aunties and uncles, cousins and grandparents. As soon as he knew that I was seeing someone (Leroy), he stopped paying any maintenance, but you were still regularly spending time with him so I did nothing, even though it meant I got further into debt. His maintenance the first year we were in London consisted of him paying the before and after school care for you both. Now I had to pay that as well as everything else. I, of course, assumed that your dad was still going to AA and that he was not drinking because this is what he told me. You did not tell me differently at the time and neither did your dad's family.

Looking back on the two years in London, I wonder what kind of a parent I was. The move down to London, initially, really distressed you both. I uprooted you from your school and your friends. I hope that you can somehow see that my dad's death triggered something in me that caused me to move to London. I really wanted you both to have a relationship with your own father and I did not want you to feel as alone in the world as I did. Your grandparents were lovely people who really cared for the two of you and often they made up the slack for your dad who was not always able to care for you. You really got on well with one of your aunties and her children. She was also a single parent and the two of us often got together with you kids. Of course, after I started dating Leroy, it became more difficult for us to meet up, as there were obviously divided loyalties.

I can honestly say that I had your best interests at heart, but I was also struggling to cope with my own feelings of inadequacy. My own childhood had no stability. My parents were constantly on the move and during my formative years, I lived in five different countries. By the time I was fourteen, I had lived in Congo, England, and Zambia, back to Congo, South Africa, and Kenya, and had moved school six times. From the age of four onward, I rarely lived at home with my parents although they were a constant presence in my life through letters and holiday visits. We lived for one year in England, during which time I had my tenth birthday. Even that year was not really normal family life as my father was away for most of the time as he had something like three hundred and fifty preaching engagements in different parts of the United Kingdom.

At the time, when I was growing up, I just accepted all the moving around. I felt sad and lonely at boarding school, but I don't remember telling my parents how I felt. I enjoyed living at home in England and I also liked the fact that I was home every night when we lived in South Africa, but I didn't enjoy going to school there for the first year as I was quite badly bullied. Again, I don't remember telling anyone about this at the time. The second year we were there, it got a bit better as I was moved into the top class and there were some kids there that I got on with. What I am trying to explain is that I had no roots. There was nowhere that I really felt was home, and I always seemed to be on the move. Even when I married your dad, we seemed to move house a lot. We were married for nine years and lived in seven different houses/apartments.

My wish as a little girl was to have a little white cottage somewhere where I would stay forever without moving. It would be surrounded by a beautiful garden with lots of sweet smelling flowers and green grass. I would live there in peace with my husband and we would never move. As I got older I had lots of other dreams. After I had you two, I dreamt that when you got older and were teenagers that my house would be full of your friends who would be drinking tea, eating sandwiches, laughing, and playing board games—just happy to have somewhere to socialize and be with other young people. They would all really like me and be appreciative of the fact that I was happy to have hordes of teenagers in my house. I even envisaged that Daniel would marry one of Sally's friends and Sally would marry one of Daniel's friends. This is what I wanted, but it is not what happened.

You see, I had a kind of dream, but I did not have a plan. Because I have always lived my life one day at a time, since I can remember, I haven't really had a plan. I just get up in the morning and do my day. Life has just kind of happened to me. There are great things about living one day at a time, and it is in fact the only way that I can cope with life, but it does mean that it is hard to have a game plan.

I remember reading once about Victoria Beckham that at a young age she decided that she was going to be famous. She didn't have a fabulous voice, but it was passable; she took singing lessons and entered singing competitions. She had a plan, stuck to it and, boy, is she famous. Even now, I don't really have a plan. I have absolutely no idea where I will be living one year from now. I still live one day at a time. When we moved to London, I truly believed that that was where I was going to stay until at least you two had finished high school and gone to university. (Yes, university—I had this notion that you would both leave high school with fantastic grades and that all the universities in the country would be anxious to have you on board because you were both so brilliant. So that is one thing I have always believed in—your talents.)

But I digress; the reality of your lives was that you were living with a mum who had no roots and who kept moving and were coping with an alcoholic father and stepdad.

Know that I loved you above all else, nonetheless.

Mum

xxxx

LETTER 8

Back to Stoke on Trent

Dear Daniel and Sally,

Yet, another move was in the cards. The renters in Stoke were not paying and I also had a mortgage on the flat in London. Leroy had been in the process of buying a flat in Egham, Surrey, when we met so there we were paying three mortgages. I was paying two and Leroy was paying one. We decided that in the New Year, we would put all three properties on the market and live in the one that was taking the longest to sell.

Leroy's flat in Egham, Surrey, sold the day he put it on the market; the flat in South East London took a couple of weeks to sell so we were on the move back to Stoke again. I had hoped that Leroy's flat in Egham would sell and the house in Stoke would sell because I really did not want to move back to Stoke. It seemed like admitting defeat: "Look at me. I am back. It didn't work out and now here I am, back where I started."

I also did not want to move back because I did not want to unsettle you both again as it seemed that it had taken nearly a year for you to get over the initial move to London. In addition, I knew that visits to your dad or with your dad's family would be infrequent due to the cost of travelling to London. I remember talking to Leroy about the realities of moving to Stoke-on-Trent. I explained that it would mean that you both would not see that much of your dad and his family, which would mean that you would be with us all the time. I knew life would be very different there, as we three had lived there before. London is a large busy city. It has its downside: more crime, more crowding, and more pollution. But it also has its upside: better public transportation, better restaurants, and better job prospects, to name just a few.

My tenants in Stoke were still not paying their rent and were leading me on with stories of how they were looking to buy the house from me at the end of their tenancy, as they were obviously aware that I had put it on the market. I then heard that they had bought another house locally and they moved out at the end of their tenancy. I was furious; they obviously had money to put a deposit on a house and were financially secure enough to get a mortgage, but just didn't like paying their rent to me!

The most sensible thing to do seemed to be to move back to live in the house in Stoke-on-Trent, so Leroy and I both started applying for jobs near Stoke. On top of it being the slowest to sell, it was also the most suitable place to live in as a family. It had three decent-sized bedrooms, an extra toilet and washbasin downstairs, beautiful country views out the back, good neighbors and a decent-sized garden. I went for an interview for a Head of Department's job in Cheshire, which was about thirty minutes drive from the house. I got the job and so we were set to move. Leroy was working for a large company, which subcontracted him out to various other companies and he got a re-location to Northampton. It wasn't exactly commutable and he would have to stay there during the week, but it was nearer to Stoke than London.

I thought that both of you would be very excited to move back to our old house in Stoke and get back together with your old friends, but found that you, Daniel, had settled in London and really wanted to stay there, and although you, Sally, seemed all right about going back, I knew that you would really miss your grandparents, aunties, and cousins. I must say that your dad did not want you to move away and even offered for Daniel to remain in London and live with him. I decided that I would give you, Daniel, the choice of staying with him or moving back up to Stoke with us. It was really touch-and-go as to what you would decide and you did not finally make up your mind to move back to Stoke until just before we moved.

It was whilst we were making plans to move and after I got the job in Cheshire that I found out that I was pregnant, so I felt there was an even greater need for us to live in a house and not an upstairs flat. After the awful start to the New Year, Leroy's drinking seemed to settle down for a while and we had a pleasant visit from my sister and her family in January along with a holiday in the Lake District with Leo in March. After the holiday in the Lake District, we drove Leo back up to Scotland and although Leroy had not drunk any alcohol whilst we were in the Lake District, he sure made up for it when we got to Scotland and started another bender. From then on, his drinking became heavier and heavier. The binges got longer and the time between the binges got shorter. Finally, not long before we moved in July, he actually joined AA in London whilst still continuing to drink. By this time, I was a few months pregnant and very apprehensive about the move, the new job, and about life in general. I really did not know how I was going to cope with a new baby, new job, drinking husband, and you two approaching your teenage years. It would be back to the situation where you did not have much contact with your dad or his family, but I soldiered on and kept all my problems to myself, trying to put on a brave face to family and friends. On the inside, I was feeling more and more anxiety and trepidation about the future.

To top it all, I was also told by the hospital that the baby I was carrying was more than likely going to be a Down's syndrome baby, so all the while I was wondering how I was going to cope with that eventuality. Naturally because of what I had been through at age eighteen, there was no way I would consider having an abortion as I strongly felt that this was wrong. Leroy was always convinced that the baby I was carrying would not have Down's syndrome and was always very positive about how we would cope with having a baby, as he was just so excited that I was pregnant (when he wasn't drinking). When I raised concerns about childcare after the baby was born, he reassured me that we would hire a nanny who would also be able to help me with caring for you two before and after school. He seemed so positive that everything would be okay and that reassured me for a while.

So shortly after the end of the school year, we moved back to Stoke-on-Trent, and I now know that it was not something that either of you wanted to do and that yet again you were unsettled. We mothers have a lot of guilt to deal with, and looking back, I feel guilty that you moved around so much when you were young yet at the time it seemed the right thing to do. In fact, it seemed like it was the only thing and most sensible thing to do. Like I said before, I had no game plan; life just happened to me and I lived one day at a time. It seemed to be the only way I could cope. One of the schools I went to had the Latin motto *Carpe diem* or something like that and I took it to heart; it is translated to mean, "seize the day." So the way I interpreted it was: An opportunity arises and you seize it—you haven't planned it—you seize it as it might not come your way again.

I guess I have a little bit of the adventurer inside of me and although on the outside I might seem sensible and calm, I am a little bit of a risk taker and sometimes throw caution to the wind. I hope at least that you do not regret all your past and can embrace the fact that you saw a bit of life. I hope that it opens your eyes to the endless possibilities that life offers each of us. Each lifestyle has its advantages; moving around can produce resilience and is the antidote to the small-mindedness that sometimes occurs in people who remain all their lives in one place.

As always, I loved and cherished you both. A new chapter was unfolding in our lives and it was to be a rocky ride, but we did not know just how rocky at the time. It is a good job that we humans don't know what lies ahead of us as we might give up too soon.

Love,

Mum

xxxx

LETTER 9

Off to Your Dad's and Back Again

Dear Daniel,

Well, here is really where you and Sally's lives took a different turn. Adolescence came to you and I did not really have the skills to cope with the escalation of testosterone in the house or whatever it was. I can't say that you changed overnight; it was more that you became increasingly difficult to parent.

Yet, again, I investigated the best schools in the area and wanted to send you to a school just over the county boundary in Cheshire. Although our address was Stoke-on-Trent, we were living just on the border between Staffordshire and Cheshire. I appealed and got you into the school as I was teaching in Cheshire and the holidays were different. This was cause enough for you to be given a place in the Cheshire school. Quite a few of your old friends from primary school were at the school, so I thought that you would be happy and fit in well. I started my new job and you started your new school, Sally went back to Year Six in her old school, which was only a five-minute walk from the house. I was nearly six months pregnant and feeling it, especially as I had had an injury to my left arm and could not use it for a couple of months due to a badly administered blood test.

Looking back, you must have been feeling really disorientated and disgruntled. I remember getting a phone call from your head of year on the first day of school. Apparently you did not like the class he had put you in, so refused to enter the class. He had told you that if you did not go in, you would have to sit in his office all day. To his surprise you said okay and plunked yourself down in his office. This, of course, was not what he was expecting and was also highly inconvenient to him, so he rang me. The upshot of the conversation was that you had refused to do anything he asked and had insisted that you would only listen to me. I asked you over the phone to give it a shot and see how things turned out and you then agreed to go to class.

I can't remember if you were eventually moved to the class of your choice, but in any case, you seemed to settle in well. You joined the football team and ended up being joint top scorer for Year Eight. In fact, you seemed to be good at everything that you put your hand to. Sporting wise, you were co-coordinated and fit. Academically, you had no problems at all and it looked as though you would have a promising school career. There were only a couple of small problems: you did not accept authority and you craved popularity with the other students. You loved to be the class clown and did not care whether or not you got into trouble. Apart from this, you seemed to be okay. Leroy was working away all week so basically, it was back to how it had been before we moved to London. His grandmother died and after spending ten weeks without a drink, he commenced the longest binge of his life. You guys did not seem to notice, but from when I picked him up from the train station on a Friday evening until I took him back on a Sunday evening, he drank. It eventually got so bad that he could no longer do the commute and rang in sick. From then on (beginning of October, I think), he remained at home. As he spent most of his time drinking upstairs in the bedroom, life continued as normal around him. I, of course, was insanely worried, but said nothing.

In the middle of October just before he was due to go to Florida with Leo, he agreed to go to AA again. It was a start, but he did not stop drinking. At this point, I took maternity leave as I could no longer cope with going to work and I was eight weeks off having the baby. Of course, as you now know, Leroy was hospitalized on his return from Florida having nearly drunk himself to death on the trip. I told you and Sally that he had suffered food poisoning because I was too embarrassed and ashamed to tell you that it was alcoholic poisoning. This is also what I told everyone else.

Looking back, what a coward I was! Truth is always better than fiction. This is really one thing I regret, as I truly believe that honesty is crucial in relationships; all trust is based on honesty. Telling the truth at this point would have saved a lot of heartache later, but part of the problem with alcoholics and drug abusers is that they deny there is a problem and often families become complicit in this denial. This is certainly the case with me; I acknowledged the problem privately and at Al Anon meetings, but denied it to family and friends. Partly this is because at Al Anon, we were encouraged to protect the anonymity of the alcoholic so therefore the program encourages complicit denial in a roundabout kind of way.

The trip to Florida became Leroy's rock bottom and from there on in he started his recovery. To this day he has never taken another drink and this in itself is nothing short of a miracle.

I digress again; can you see, Daniel, how abuse of alcohol ruins the fabric of family life? It is the hidden monster in the house, lurking to attack at every turn. In the meantime, you got on with your life. We had a few run-ins; the rebellion was starting to show. In London, you had started to steal money from us and this continued. Of course, you will now realize that I was actually very short of money, so although some of your theft went unnoticed, there was one time when you stole some money from my purse that I had put aside to put in a collection at my uncle's funeral. Usual story: you denied it, I pursued, and eventually the money was recovered from a girl who lived down the road from us. (You had given it to her for safekeeping.) I wanted to frighten you with the reality of theft and took you to the police station. It turns out that you wanted a particular kind of yoyo. Unbeknown to you, I had already bought you one for Christmas and it was wrapped up in my cupboard, but as usual you wanted it *now*. That was how it was with you; you always wanted things instantly and could not bear to wait.

Just before your thirteenth birthday, you asked me for clothes for your birthday. I told you how much money I had to spend on you and you decided what you wanted. I explained that if you spent all the money on clothes, I would not be able to take you out on your birthday as well. You just wanted the puffer jacket and a few other things so we bought them. I wanted to wrap them up and give you them on your birthday, but no, you wanted them instantly. I gave in and let you have them. Then on the day of your birthday, you were disappointed; you already had your presents and there was no outing to look forward to. I made you a cake and we all sang happy birthday, but you were very moody and unhappy. By this time Lilly had been born and was three months old. I was breastfeeding her and could not leave her with anyone for any length of time. My hands were really tied. In fact, I would have loved to go out and take you to Pizza Hut or the cinema as I was totally housebound at the time and suffering postnatal depression, but I actually could not. You did not understand. Leroy had stopped drinking and had started work again shortly after Lilly's birth, but he was working an hour and a half commute from where we lived and had the use of the car all week. Your birthday was at the weekend, but he was not confident to have Lilly for more than twenty minutes in case she started crying and he could not deal with her. She had severe eczema and breastfeeding seemed to calm her down when she was itchy and crying.

I am not sure if you remember this day, but I do, probably because it was the start of your teenage years. It left me with a very bad feeling; I felt a failure as a mother to you. I ended up taking you to the video shop to rent a movie as that was just about all I could afford to do time-wise and money-wise. We had an argument in the video shop because you chose videos that I would not allow you to see. It was a constant battle between you and me; you always wanted to push the boundaries and always did. Like all kids, you needed a father's firm, but kind discipline as well as a mother's care. You needed both a mum and a dad and most of the time you only had a mum. I really felt like I was losing control.

The year progressed and I became more and more tied to the house with Lilly. I could not go back to work as planned because I could not find suitable childcare for her. The nanny idea did not materialize mostly because it was exorbitantly expensive, but also because we did not have the room for a live-in nanny or even an *au pair*. I was now on unpaid maternity leave and had no money of my own. Leroy and I had not come to the point in our marriage where we shared everything so I was totally reliant on him giving me money and he was finding the reality of running a household to be a complete financial shock. He emerged out of his life with booze to find that he was married with a wife about to give birth, two stepchildren and a son of his own who lived in Scotland. For the first time in twenty-five years of drinking, he had no crutch, no escape from reality.

Sally, of course, was also approaching puberty and was beginning to be cheeky and rebellious and you two were continuing to fight with each other both for my time and affection, but also just because you got on each other's nerves. It was in this scenario that Leo came to stay with us for a couple of weeks at the end of the school year. Schools in Scotland break up earlier than the ones in England so he was on holiday earlier than you were. Leroy was working so I was in charge yet again. I had made plans to return to work at the start of the following school year and we had bought a small Peugeot 106 as a second car so that I would be able to get to work.

You and Leo seemed to get on very well. You spent a lot of time out and about in the neighborhood, often hanging out with a few other boys that you knew. A neighbor I had never met before came knocking one day (hot on your heels) and ranted and raved at me about how the two of you were the worst boys she had ever come across. I could not get to the bottom of what had gone on; it seemed to consist of a few minor pranks (knocking on doors and running away) and swearing. I told you off and told you not to go near her house again, but that was it. I didn't really take it too seriously. Toward the end of Leo's stay, he asked me if you could return home with him for a couple of weeks and stay with his mum. I was very hesitant about allowing this and had grave reservations as I did not know Leo's mum very well, but you both were really keen. In the end, I was just plain tired and agreed. You went back with Leo and it was arranged that Leroy and I would drive up to Scotland the next week and pick you up.

Well, what a disaster that was. It is a decision I will always regret. If I remember correctly, we drove up to Scotland and back in one day and it was a good four-hour drive each way. We left very early in the morning with Sally and Lilly who was by then only eight months old. We met up with you at Leroy's parent's house when we got there and told you that we were leaving to come back at 6:00 p.m. You and Leo were very elusive and kept disappearing. Leo's mum rang to speak to Leroy and he went down to see her. It appeared that you had both been in trouble with the police and she wanted him to do something about it. Something about running over roofs in the middle of the night. I never got to the bottom of that one! We packed the car to return home, got Lilly changed, fed, and ready for the long journey and at 6:00 p.m., there was no sign of you anywhere. We rang Leo's mum; neither of you were there. She suggested that we look in the park. We went down to the park and some kids there said that you had been there, but had left. Finally after searching for a few hours, Leroy decided that we would return back to Stoke without you. We gave some money to Leroy's mum and asked her to put you on the train to Stoke-on-Trent the next day. She agreed to put you up for the night and take you to the train station the next day. Again I was a coward. I did not want to leave you there and was in fact very worried as to your whereabouts. Leroy was sure that you were safe; he was just very angry that you had gone missing with Leo and thought that the two of you were deliberately messing him about.

To be fair, we faced a very long drive back, had a very long day and had a baby in the car. I actually felt like vomiting I was so anxious about the whole situation, but Leroy was so angry that I could not persuade him to wait any longer. It is so easy in retrospect; maybe I should have stood my ground and insisted on waiting until you turned up— maybe not. Would things have turned out any differently—who knows? Once we were well and truly on our way, my mobile phone rang and it was you. You screamed obscenities down the phone at me and demanded that I return to pick you up. I could not return, as I was not driving. I explained that I would meet you from the train the next day. On the one hand, I was relieved that you were in fact safe, on the other, I was now frightened at the effect this would have on our relationship. I now had two very angry people to deal with: Leroy and you. (In fact, three very angry people, as Sally was also very angry although I am not sure if she was angry with Leroy, you, me, or all of us.)

When I got home, I was exhausted and spent another sleepless night with Lilly. The next day, I figured that everyone would have calmed down and that you especially would be very repentant and sorry for messing us about. I thought that being left behind and having to spend the night at Leroy's mum's followed by a train journey home would have given you time to think, be sorry and that you would have been taught a valuable lesson. On the contrary, you were even angrier than you had been the night before. When I met you, you were seething with rage. There was no shred of remorse or regret in you. All I was met with was a tirade of abuse about Leroy. It turned out that during the week you spent with Leo's mum, she had done a very good job of turning you completely against Leroy. She had told you that he had said that he hated you and Sally because you were English and that he would slit your throats if England beat Scotland in a football game. I could not believe my ears. He had apparently said this the previous year before Lilly was born and he had gone to Scotland to see Leo. It was the time that I had gone with him, but had taken a return flight back to London, as he was so drunk when we got off the plane, he just wanted to carry on drinking. She also made you believe that he was likely having an affair because she got it out of you that he was going out on a Thursday night. She asked you if you knew where he was going and if I went with him. When you said that he went on his own, she got you to believe that he was probably cheating on me.

Here I was in a car with a boy that was seething with anger, resentment, with no sign of remorse and who was now openly against his new stepdad. Looking back, I should not have let you go and stay with Leo and his mum. It was not right at that time. She was not in a good place emotionally and was finding Leo tough to bring up. To be honest, I do not really know what was going through her mind, or whether she herself had been drinking when she told you these things. It may be that you misunderstood some of the things that she said. I really do not know. All I know is the result that it had on you and it was this visit that was the turning point in our relationship. I have always been such a coward and hated confrontation so much that I was scared of bringing you home and confronting Leroy with everything that you said. I knew that he was expecting you back home eating humble pie, showing remorse for the way you had messed us around. I knew you were not sorry and could not see that you had done anything wrong; instead you were very angry with both of us for leaving you behind and making you come back on the train. It did not seem that there was any answer to this one.

I knew that you were missing your dad and all your relatives in London and I thought it would benefit you if you went and spent some time with him over the summer. You seemed keen on this idea so I contacted your dad who was also keen. Leroy thought it was a good idea because I told him what had been said about him and he denied talking about you and Sally that way. He did not want me to tell you that he was an alcoholic and that he was going to AA on Thursday nights, but I had already told you this in the car on the way back from the train station so that you would understand why he went out and realize that he was not having an affair.

What happened next was not really what I had planned. You did indeed go to your dad's for the summer, but with a curious twist of events, you ended up staying there for a year. Your dad really did want you to go and live with him. He had, however, sold his one-bedroom flat and was in the process of buying somewhere else in London. It was in a less desirable area, but could still accommodate you. He wanted you to stay longer than the summer, and to be honest, I thought it was a good idea. I was finding the tension in the house between you and Leroy very unmanageable and thought it would be best for everyone, so I encouraged the idea. I thought that you would just go back to your old school and slot back in with your old friends and enjoy living near your cousins and grandparents.

One of the stipulations that your dad had given me about you going back to stay with him was that he did not want you to make visits back up to Stoke as he felt it might unsettle you and make you want to come back and live with me. He stipulated that you were not to make any visits until Christmastime. He would not even allow you to come back and get your things. You had initially gone down with a suitcase, but obviously needed more of your personal possessions. He made me promise that you could stay there for at least a year.

So the situation between you and me and between Leroy and you was not sorted out. It was merely pushed aside and not dealt with. I was really sad that you were going to live with your dad, but was also relieved as I was having trouble coping with life in general. I thought that your dad had a responsibility toward you and also I had no idea that he was drinking again. I knew that you needed a positive male role model in your life and hoped that your dad would rise to the challenge. He had always seemed to have a special relationship with you and I thought the responsibility of having you to live with him would bring out the best in him. You were not a baby and were of an age where I thought you and your dad could form a good bond. I could see that Leroy was not going to be able to rise to the challenge of being that role model. He would provide for you, but would expect respect and obedience and he actually did not want to replace your dad. The thing he feared the most was that you would say, "F—O—, you are not my dad."

He has a very short fuse and does not cope with confrontation in any other way than with increased confrontation. He did not want to lose it with you for fear of the consequences. I guess he was always afraid that he would say or do things that he later regretted. On top of all this, he was in his first year of not drinking and only just managing that one day at a time.

Dear Daniel, this decision to send you to your dad's for a year is one that I regret deeply. Who knows how things would have turned out if I had faced the undercurrents of anger and mistrust in the house and stood my ground? Deep down, I feared that your mistrust of him and his short fuse would end in a huge confrontation with Leroy leaving me. This would not be a winning situation even for you as you still would not have a positive male role model and now Lilly would be fatherless, too. Many of my decisions were based on this fear. The trouble with me is that I can usually see a problem from more than one angle; this makes life complicated because I don't have a clear vision of what needs to be done in a certain situation. I guess deep down one of my goals was to preserve my marriage, as I did not want to get divorced again. Having gone through it once and having always believed that marriage is for life, I wanted to do everything in my power to keep this one alive. However, life is not as simple as that; mostly I have just lived one day at a time. My job in this instance and in many others was what I call *damage limitation.* That is, the decision that I can make that will bring about the least damage to members of the family. I could not now only be thinking of consequences for you and Sally; I also had to take Lilly into consideration. I also saw hope in my marital relationship as Leroy had stopped drinking and I could see what a great father he was to Lilly. He absolutely doted on her. His whole world revolved around her. I had never seen this from your dad. I hoped that by going to your dad's you would gain something; I hoped that it would enable Leroy to get more used to life without alcohol and that somehow if and when you came back to live with us that life would be better—magically!

Unfortunately, you did not get back into the same school you had left. I do not know what your dad did, but you ended up not being at school for months on end. You had no phone in the house and mobile phones were not common then. I basically lost contact with you for weeks on end. I wrote you letters and sent you *Stoke City* magazines, but had very little response back. Eventually your dad got you enrolled in another school in London near to where he was now living. It was not a great school and none of your previous friends went there. You have not told me much about it, but I don't think it was a great experience for you. I do know that living with your dad was proving to be very different from spending the weekend with him. He had returned to drinking and was becoming quite violent when drunk. You never told me any of this at the time. My first inkling that something was wrong was when you came back on your Christmas visit. Your dad and I did a swap. I took Sally down to see him and he met me at the train station with you. I took you back up with me and then when your visit was over, I took you back down to London by train and he then met me with Sally, who I accompanied back up to Stoke. As usual, I paid for all the train fares and made all the arrangements. It was on that train journey that you actually opened up to me about what living with your dad had been like for you.

On the visit, I had been very strict with you and Leroy and I had not allowed you out at night at all. There was one exception: New Year's Eve 1999, the dawn of the new century. Leroy and I had been invited to a joint AA/Al Anon party and you asked us if you could go out with some of your friends from your old school and stay the night with one of them. Selfishly, because we wanted to go to the party, we took our eyes off the ball so to speak and allowed you to go to your party so that we could go to ours. After all, we were welcoming in the year 2000. Sally was, of course, down in London with her dad and grandparents and Lilly could come along with us as she was still small enough to go to sleep in her car chair, which could be carried out of the car and then used as a rocker in the house.

To cut to the chase, unbeknown to us you got drunk that night and with a couple of others vandalized the local primary school. This act came back to roost later in the year after you had returned to your dad's, and it was added to your police record. By this time, you had been in trouble with the police several times over minor offences, including stealing from us. Most of the offences were related to vandalism and resisting authority. However, at the time we did not know about it and so all in all we deemed the visit a success. There were no confrontations between you and Leroy and things seemed to go quite well. I was happy.

On the train journey to London when we were about halfway there, you suddenly turned to me and said, "Mum, I would eat s—- to come back and live with you."

To say I was shocked was an understatement, as you had not indicated once during your stay that you hated it at your dad's. Then it all came pouring out: your dad was drinking again and when he was drunk he was sometimes violent; if you disobeyed him in the slightest or did anything that annoyed him and he had been drinking, he would hit you. Of course, the next morning he would not remember what he had done. I told you that you should return straight home. We would collect Sally and come back together. Then you seemed to change your mind and you said, "Mum, I can't come back now as I promised my dad that I would live with him for at least a year. Can I come back at the end of the year?"

Of course, I said, "Yes."

I then asked you repeatedly if you would return earlier and you said that you could not.

So there you stayed until the end of the school year. Life carried on back in Stoke, but underneath it all, I was very worried about you and what effect living at your dad's was having on you. In the meantime, I was very busy with Lilly and Sally and started back at work after a long maternity leave. We eventually put Lilly in a local nursery, and I dropped her off on my way to work. It was now clear to us that eczema was not her only problem as she could not tolerate cow's milk and we discovered she had an allergy to eggs. She was constantly breaking out in rashes and hives and sometimes her whole body would flare up. We then discovered that she was allergic to grass, cats, and various scents. It was a constant struggle trying to keep her comfortable and deal with her often-unpredictable allergic reactions, which ranged from vomiting and diarrhea to extreme redness and swelling all over her body. I had to completely reassess how to care for her.

In the spring, we had a trip to Malta as a family and you were supposed to come along, but Stoke City got into the Auto Windshield Cup Final and you decided that you would rather stay and watch that match than come on holiday with us. Your reason was a good one as it was one of the last games to be played at the original Wembley Stadium and you were a huge Stoke City fan. I can see now that watching your team play at the iconic stadium was more important to you than a holiday in Malta, but at the time I did not understand and was very disappointed. Leroy was upset because he had already paid for your fare and accommodation, but fortunately they let us change the tickets and Nana came in your place.

We also had visits from the police during the year and that is when we discovered that you had been involved in the vandalism on New Year's Eve. This was something that you were going to have to face when you returned from London.

I look back on these years and I must admit I do have regrets. Sometimes, these regrets overwhelm me and I have spent a lot of time wondering about the what-ifs. What if you had not gone to London for the year with your dad? What if I had not allowed you to go and stay with Leo and his mum? What if I had been open about Leroy's drinking problem? What if I had been braver in my parenting?

You see when you came back from your dad's is when it all seemed to go terribly wrong.

There had been some good things about your stay in London. I had bought you a tennis racquet when you went down to London and your dad enrolled you in some tennis coaching lessons. Apparently you were very good at tennis and this is something you really wanted to continue. I was happy that you had found another sport that you liked and wanted to encourage you to continue. I just never got it together; the co-ordination of finding out about the lessons, enrolling you, and getting you there were just too much for me. Leroy was still pretty insistent that I was always available for Lilly, particularly now that she was developing all the allergies. Unbeknown to you, I was also pregnant and during the next few months, Sally took the limelight as things erupted in an ugly way between her and Leroy. You returned home in August and by Christmas of that year, Sally had been to stay at Nana's for seven weeks (September/October), I had a car crash (September), we went to Scot-

land for a week (October), I had a miscarriage, Leroy had left me
(November) and returned (November) and we had moved to a bigger
house nearer to your school (December). You had started back at the
school in Cheshire and seemed fairly happy to be back. We had forbidden you to drink after the New Year's Eve episode, which had been
fueled by drinking. You did not appear to be drinking and I could not
smell alcohol on you, but something was going on; you seemed to sleep
all the time you were home at the weekends after going out with
friends, but then teenagers need more sleep, don't they? Of course, it all
became clear when it transpired that you had started to smoke weed,
but I did not really discover that until December.

Recently, I was trying to figure out why I had not pursued the tennis
lessons for you and when I sat down and thought about it some more, I
realized it was because too much else was going on in our lives. Of
course, on top of all this, I was working full time as Head of Department in a Secondary School and was slowly drowning in paperwork.
The teaching itself I loved; the reports, marking, etc.—I just could not
keep up with. I already knew that I had let the school down badly by
having an extended maternity leave just following my appointment. I
was supposed to be revamping an ailing department and I basically was
not there. Now that I was back, the school understandably wanted me
to go full steam ahead, but I just was not up to it. In reality, I was suffering from depression, triggered by a form of post-natal depression that
had been worsened by my personal circumstances, particularly living
with alcoholism, dealing with turbulent teenagers (including a stepson),
having a baby with allergies, and trying to pay back money debts.

So I guess what I am trying to say is, sorry about the tennis lessons.
Who knows if things would have turned out differently if you had pursued this at that time; maybe smoking weed would not have become
your favorite pastime, but then again, maybe it would. Maybe, also, this
is the reason that I now try to pursue every interest that your younger
brother and sister have. I want them to find their niche, have a passion,
and not turn to alcohol or drugs for their enjoyment. I want them to
have music lessons, swimming lessons, tennis lessons, and ballet lessons, if that is what they want to do. I am trying to help them find
enjoyment and fun in life. The ballet, tennis, and swimming lessons
have already fallen by the wayside, although both of them are compe-
tent swimmers, but the music seems to be an ongoing interest so whilst
I can, I am encouraging them to pursue it. It may seem to be unfair to
you, but I guess we learn from our mistakes. Also, I am in a better

financial position now. I did what I could at the time you were growing up and that is just how it is.

Being fair is not necessarily giving everyone the same thing; I am learning that it is giving everyone what he or she needs. In a family situation, this means that each child is treated as an individual. Your younger brother in particular gets far more spent on him than you ever did, but he is autistic. He gets speech therapy, occupational therapy, and behavior modification. We have a trampoline; he has a beanbag and a rocking chair and a fan on all night to help him sleep. He also gets a lion's share of my time and attention, but think about it: would you rather be you, or would you rather have to contend with his disability all your life? I know Callum would rather be who he is, as he is beginning to embrace his differences, but I also know you would also rather be you. You never needed all these therapies.

I love you and always have. What I have lacked in parenting skills, I have made up for in persevering in my love for you and never giving up on you even when things seemingly became hopeless.

Mum

xxxx

LETTER 10

Off to Your Nana's and Back Again

Dear Sally,

Well, this is going to be a hard letter to write; there is no doubt about that. This stay at your Nana's has become a turning point in your life. I have been writing to your brother, Daniel, about my cowardice and here again, in this situation, it surfaces. I hate confrontation in any form and obviously you can't be alive and not have confrontations, differences of opinion, and difficult situations. I have had my fair share of difficult situations, but flight not fight has been my initial response.

If I have gone over what happened a hundred times I have gone over it a thousand times in my head. After moving back up to Stoke-on-Trent, you went back to your old primary school and hooked up with your old friends in the neighborhood and at school. Leroy stopped drinking and I had Lilly. There were a few ups and downs. I noticed a change in you after Lilly was born and could not help feeling sorry for you as you saw how besotted Leroy was with Lilly. His whole life seemed to revolve around her and her well-being. I know that you probably coveted his doting on her and wished that your own father would be the same with you.

We were back in our old house and at first this sufficed. Lilly had a cot in our bedroom and you and Daniel had your old bedrooms back. It must have been good to have some space back as you had such a tiny room in London. It seemed to me to be a better place to bring up you kids. You could actually go out of the house and I was not afraid that you would be mugged. We went back to visiting Nana in Wales and you seemed to get on well with Leroy, although after Lilly's birth not so well as before. You were always asking if you could push Lilly round the neighborhood in her pushchair to show all your friends and Leroy would not allow it. Maybe this is one of the things I should have fought for. Who knows? Daniel was in Secondary School and you did not hang out with him very much. Mostly you went around with girls and boys from school.

You were starting to become "cheeky" with me. I remember one occasion (Bonfire night) when you wanted to go and look at the local bonfire on the field opposite the house. I had never allowed you and

Daniel to go when we lived there previously as all the locals threw their old tat on a big pile and then this was burnt on Bonfire night. The pile was dangerous and I was sure that the fire would be full of toxic fumes as people dumped their old mattresses, furniture, and general rubbish. Looking back, I guess I was a bit of a stick in the mud. There were certain things that I just would not allow and others where I was not strict at all. It must have seemed very appealing as a child to see the flames go up and feel the heat of the fire on a cold autumn night and feel the excitement of the night with all the other kids from the neighborhood running around. I am a bit scared of fire and was also seven months pregnant at the time. Leroy had finally stopped drinking after nearly killing himself on the trip to Florida and had only been home from hospital for a week. I was totally shattered emotionally and physically, so when you started pestering me about going to see the bonfire I was in no mood for giving in. I could not understand why you were even asking because I had never allowed you to go before; however, you persisted and in the end screamed obscenities at me because I said no.

That was it; I completely lost it and slapped you across the face. You ran upstairs continuing to scream abuse at me and slammed the door to your bedroom. My memory does not serve me well as to what happened next. I know I did not give in and let you go out and I thought that I ended up throwing cold water over you, but I am not sure if it was on this occasion or another. So you can see, my dear girl, things were not always rosy between us, but on the whole, I felt we were very close and of course, I loved you dearly. This occasion is in fact the only occasion I can really remember slapping you, although I am sure you will remember others. Generally, you were a very obedient child and a very loving one, but the hormones were starting to kick in and as we all know when that happens, sometimes youngsters start to kick out at the people nearest to them. I feel I have always copped it from you, as you know that my love for you is unconditional and therefore I am probably a safe person to let rip with. I don't know. In a way, my relationship with you is unique above all my children as I really have been a single parent to you all your life. You never really bonded with your own father (not your fault at all) and Leroy never was the stepfather you thought he might become. He has provided for you; he has cared for you, but he has not been a *daddy* to you. Some men just don't know what they are missing out on when they don't care for or connect with their children. I am sad for you that you have missed out in this way with your own dad. I hope that it will not color your opinion of all men, as there are many good ones out there. I know that your granddad, on your dad's side, was a great role model for you and you felt and received lots of love from both him and Granny. I also feel that you have a very special relationship with my mum, your nana, which brings me to the topic of this letter.

For the second year we were back in Stoke-On-Trent, Daniel was down living with your dad and you started high school. One day, I discovered that you were smoking, quite by accident. Leroy and I decided to go and do a bit of shopping at the local supermarket and as we parked behind it, we saw you walking in the park with some of your friends, bold as brass smoking a cigarette. I was surprised, but not shocked as both Leroy and I were smokers. I had suspected that Daniel was smoking, but you both used to give me so many lectures about my own smoking that it did kind of take me by surprise. Looking back now, I am surprised at my own reaction. Most parents would have given their child a lambasting for underage smoking and would have punished them in some way. I don't recall doing this at all. I just told you that I had seen you smoking so you were not to deny it. I also started to keep a closer watch on my own cigarettes as I had noticed that there always seemed to be less in there than I thought there should be. That was it. You see, I was suffering from depression and was taking anti-depressants so I never got excited about anything; holidays did not excite me, nothing really did, and conversely, nothing really shocked me either. I did not have the energy to be angry. I was just surviving day to day and hardly had the energy for that.

Your friendship groups seemed to change, but on the whole you seemed to be fine. You had a few problems with a couple of the girls in the neighborhood, but would not really tell me what they were; instead, you just seemed to hide behind me when we went shopping locally. The house was calmer because Daniel was away at your dad's so there was no arguing between the two of you. You and Leo spent quite a bit of holiday time together that year, both in Malta and up caravanning in the Lake District and you seemed to get on well.

When it was decided that Daniel was returning, Leroy and I decided that we needed to have four bedrooms. I wanted Lilly to move out of our bedroom. The natural solution would have been to make you and Lilly share a room, but there was a huge age difference, and also Leroy said he would be uncomfortable going in and playing with Lilly or putting her to bed if she shared a room with you. You were twelve and starting to need your own space and privacy and you were not his natural daughter. We decided to convert the biggest bedroom—yours—into two smaller bedrooms. The builder told us that it would be easier to make the bedrooms by also adding a small hallway along one end of the bedroom and we decided to make this into a computer space for Leroy. There was only one problem: The telephone point that we would need to use for the Internet was in one of the proposed two new bedrooms. We gave you first choice of bedrooms and you chose the room with the telephone point. I tried to dissuade you from your choice as I explained that it would mean that Leroy would have to come in and out of the room to connect his computer when needed and that there would then be a wire across your floor. You were adamant you wanted that room and would not mind about the cable as long as Leroy knocked before entering the room so that you could cover up if you were dressing, or ask him to wait. This was, of course, in the days before we had broadband so all our Internet use was dial up. I was uneasy, but gave in.

The arrangement seemed to be working well at first. Daniel came back to live and moved into his old room. I moved Lilly out of my bedroom and into one of the two new rooms. Leroy moved his computer into the small hallway. There did not seem to be any problem with the telephone point access. Then one day, it all changed.

I can't remember exactly when you brought it up with me, but I remember you were very angry. It must have been on a Saturday, or a Sunday, because you told me that not only had Leroy been into your room when you were out and plugged in his computer, but that that morning you had woken up to see him plugging in his computer. You were hopping mad. You were really angry and told me to tell him that he was not allowed in your room at all. If he wanted the computer plugged in, he should knock and ask and wait for you to plug it in and if you weren't there it couldn't be plugged in. Your complaint was something along those lines. I tried to explain that when you chose the room you realized that he would need to plug in his computer, but you were not having a bar of it.

Something snapped inside of me. I am usually the mediator, the messenger especially between Daniel and you and Leroy. You talk to me about any issues you have with him and then I talk to him. It also works the other way. He talks to me about issues he has with either of you and then I talk to you. I was just plain fed up with being the cushion between you so I said that you should speak to Leroy personally. I wanted you to start communicating with each other. Later in the kitchen, I told him that you wanted to speak to him about the telephone point in your bedroom and his computer. I was also in the kitchen and so was Lilly. Daniel was out on the field with some of his friends. The conversation seemed to start quite well and I felt that it would be better if you resolved the issue between the two of you.

I was wrong.

The conversation soon became a yelling match and then a swearing match. You both gave as good as you got. You told him he had no authority over you and he called your own dad names. By this time, it was too late for me to intervene; both of you had completely lost the plot. I was shaking with fear and dread at the Pandora's box that had just been opened. My legs were like jelly and my mouth was completely dry. I was holding Lilly who by this time was crying.

I told you to go upstairs to your room and Leroy yelled at you to get out of the room. Instead of going to your room, you ran out of the front door onto the field. I did not know what to do. Leroy was totally distraught and was saying that he would never go into your room again, but that you were never to come into our room again. He was in total meltdown.

I tried to calm him down and say that we would resolve the issue by putting in another telephone point, but that it would take a week or so. I went to the door, still holding Lilly in my arms, and opened it to see if I could see you, as I wanted you to come back in the house. I didn't really know what to do and I was already feeling very sick, as I was pregnant.

As I got to the door, Daniel ran in shouting, "Where is he—where is he—I'm going to get him—he's beaten Sally."

I managed to stop him in his tracks before he reached Leroy who was still in the kitchen. I assured him that there had been a huge argument, but that Leroy had not even touched you, much less hit you.

Daniel then said, "She's on the field crying and everyone is saying that Leroy beat her up."

I calmed him down and assured him again that although there had been a bad argument and lots of shouting, no one had hit anyone. I had been there the whole time in the room so I would know.

At this point, things had gone from bad to worse. I felt that the family was now standing on a precipice and that the slightest wrong move would send us all over the edge and smash us into oblivion. How would we survive this accusation? Leroy had heard the accusation. On top of the fact that he felt the computer situation was impossible, it was now being said that he was beating you up. He told me that he would have to leave, or you would have to go and live with your dad. He also said that if he stayed, we would have to sell the house and leave the neighborhood, as he would never live down the accusation that you had made even though it was not true.

Well, when I thought things could not get any worse, they did. Some of your friends started lining up at the front of the house. One came down and knocked at the door. When I opened it, she said, "Sally is on the field; she is too scared to come home."

"She has nothing to be scared of; go and tell her to come home," I replied.

They went away. Then another delegation came to the back gate and gave the same message. I gave the same reply. I was still holding Lilly in my arms and it had started to rain. The steps were slippery and I lost my footing and fell, sending Lilly flying and spraining my ankle badly. Leroy rushed out to get Lilly and help me up and your friends ran off to get you. You finally came home, but by this time, I needed to go to the hospital as I was in agony. The physical emergency took over from the argument. Our neighbors' daughter agreed to look after you and Daniel while Leroy took me to the hospital.

Sally, like I said, I am a coward who knows what I should have done at this point. You would probably say that I should have told him to leave if he wanted to. You would say that you were only a child and he was an adult and that he should not have sworn at you or said things about your own father.

Recently, I was talking to Daniel about the incident and he said, "Mum, what you should have done was say to Sally when she first complained, 'If you don't like Leroy coming into your bedroom to plug in his computer then you will have to swap bedrooms with Lilly. End of story.'"

Hey, why didn't I think of that at the time? Perfect solution! The reason I did not think of it at the time was because I was barely thinking at all, just surviving day to day. After spending ten years with one drinking alcoholic and then having a break before spending a further eighteen months with another drinking alcoholic, I, too, was in recovery mode. Leroy was no longer drinking, but was still recovering from the effects of drinking for so long. I, too, was recovering. It is a feeble excuse, but it is the only one I have.

So I am a coward, but I am also a survivor. To me, my whole aim was to save the family unit. I could not face another break up. I was pregnant again and I had a gut feeling that if we could survive the storm, the boat would not break up. Whilst at the hospital having my ankle checked out, I tried to persuade Leroy to stay and sort things out with you. He refused to talk about it. Years later and with hindsight, I now realize that Leroy had gone from meltdown to shutdown. Through discovering more about Autism, following Callum's diagnosis, and recognizing the traits in Leroy, I have learned that one of Leroy's coping mechanisms is complete shutdown. At these times he cannot talk about the situation and usually just goes to bed and will not open his eyes, speak, eat, or drink. So the fact that he managed to come with me to the hospital was amazing. Of course, hindsight reveals more about a situation than meets the eye at the time and I was certainly not aware of this then.

My mind was working overtime. I knew we all just needed time and space. I knew things would not work out with your dad, but I did contact him first. He refused to have you to even come and stay with him. Then I rang Nana, told her what had happened, and she opened her home to you. Her only stipulations were that it was only a temporary solution and also that you could not sit at her house and do nothing, so I would have to enroll you in the local high school. I knew that I had to have a solution to the dilemma and I had to have one quickly. You see, Sally, it was no longer about the telephone wire, or even indeed the argument that you and Leroy had. It was no longer about the hurtful things that had been said in the kitchen that day. It was no longer about Leroy being a grownup, and you being a girl, or about him being held accountable for swearing at you. It was now about the fact that you had allowed all the neighbors to believe that he was abusing you physically. Men have been jailed for less. Families have been torn apart and reputations lost forever. People have lost their jobs, their whole livelihood. Even though it was not true, even though you would now go out and deny it, setting the story straight, people would just assume that there is no smoke without fire.

So really, although Leroy's behavior during the argument could be said to end up being reprehensible, as being an adult he should not have sworn at you or called your dad names, but it was now not about that. It was about the lie. You can rest assured that if indeed he had even laid a finger on you, I would have asked him to leave, and if he hadn't, he would not have seen me for dust. In fact, the opposite seemed to be true and made me a little sad. He barely seemed to notice you at all; he was so besotted with Lilly. He wanted and expected me to look after you, care for you and where necessary discipline you. He deliberately never put himself into situations that would cause direct conflict between either yourself or Daniel because he was not your dad and because he did not trust his reactions in such situations. On each occasion of conflict, his solution was that he would leave. I didn't want him to leave, because I was not sure he would ever come back. Leroy leaving in this instance would have made it look like he was guilty as accused, so in this instance I felt I had no choice. I knew you would be safe at Nana's; I knew she would look after you and I knew that I would get you back as soon as I could. I loved you and did not want you to go, but I could not really tell you this at the time and I am sorry. I took the tack of least said, soonest mended. I did not have the emotional energy to engage in conversations with you that would be full of resentment and anger. So, yes, I was a coward. I did not have the fight in me.

The best solution would probably have been for us to sit down as a family and talk about what had happened and listen to each other and make a way forward, but Leroy and I were not mature enough and stable enough as a couple to do this. We should each have been allowed to vent and rage and then calm down and come to a solution, but in stepfamilies this is very hard because there is more at stake than in a biological family. (Can I say that it is also very hard in a biological family, as I am finding out with Lilly and Leroy? Teenage daughters and their fathers face a turbulent few years.) In the case of stepparents, there is a hidden rivalry between the children and the *new* parent for the affection of the biological parent. Who does this person love the most: do they love their new partner more than their children or do they love the children they already have more than their new partner? The children have the edge, as they have obviously known the parent for longer than the new partner, and the bonds of love go far deeper; on the other hand, the adults also love each other. In my case, I did not want to have another broken marriage, and I did not want to put the child from this marriage in the same position as you and Daniel, i.e., fatherless. In no way did I feel that I was abandoning you, but I now know that this is how you felt. I felt like I was putting you in a safe place whilst I sorted out things on the home front so that you could return and we could all be reunited. On that night, I was also in a lot of pain, due to my sprained ankle. Daniel had returned to live with us, and I was pregnant again. Leroy had been sober for nearly two years and I was back at work. I really wanted things to start going well for us as a family and, of course, did not want you to live with Nana forever. I could not understand why you had said that Leroy had hit you. I just did not understand what was going on in your head.

A lot of water has gone under the bridge since that day. I now know that you were completely traumatized by going to stay at your Nana's and that you felt totally abandoned by me. This is also where the difference in concepts of time comes in. As a twelve/thirteen-year-old, the seven weeks that you stayed at your Nana's seemed like an eternity to you. For me it was seven weeks. I now realize that because I knew my intention was always for you to return, I view this time as when you stayed with your Nana. I always saw it as only temporary, but you saw it as a permanent exclusion from the family. You refer to this time as when I kicked you out. I saw not communicating for a couple of weeks as time for everyone to calm down and gather themselves together and you saw it as ex-communication.

Over many years and many times, both in writing and verbally, I have expressed deep regret over your feelings at this time and have said I'm sorry for not handling the situation in a different way. At the very least, in retrospect, I should have made sure that you knew it was temporary and I should have communicated with you daily. In those days, there was no Facebook and we did not have mobile phones or broadband or Skype. I did not have e-mail. This is how I would cope if the same situation arose today and I could not face talking to someone, but needed to let that person know that I loved him or her. If I had had those means at my disposal, I would have used them. The only ways I could communicate with you were by letter or phone. I know that I wrote because I sent you a birthday card and present (a watch). I rang Nana frequently to find out how you were, but could not face talking to you because I knew I would not be able to tell you when you could come home. Of course, I also lost the baby I was carrying partly as a result of the fall I had on that day so was in total grief and agony myself.

All my apologies have not remedied your feelings about this time. I know also that Leroy has apologized in writing to you on a few occasions. After he became a Christian, he wrote you a letter apologizing and offered to take you out shopping to buy you some clothes. He knew that buying clothes would not repay you for the damage done to the relationship, but it was his way of trying to start to build a relationship with you. You refused to go with him and in the end, we all went out as a family and I gave you the money and you bought the clothes.

So here I am again addressing the situation. I do not want to make myself out to be blameless, as I clearly could have handled things in a different way, and all I want to say is that I hurt for that hurt twelve-year-old that was you, who felt so abandoned and unloved. Let me tell you again, I loved you then and I love you now. Nothing you could do could make me love you more and nothing you could do could make me love you less. You will always be my very precious daughter. I pray that one day you will be able to replace your fear of abandonment with feelings of acceptance. I cannot promise to always approve of your decisions, but I will always accept them as your decisions. I cannot promise to never disagree with your opinions, but I will recognize your right to have your own opinions. I can't say it often enough. *I will always love you.*

After physically getting over the loss of my baby, I persuaded Leroy that it was time for you to come home. I can't remember exactly, but I think that you either wrote or said to him that you were sorry for saying that he had beaten you and you came home.

He was also grieving the loss of our baby deeply, but we were trying to move on. We decided that the way to cope with the situation of thinking that the entire neighborhood believed that he was a child-beater was to move to another neighborhood, although having lost the baby, there was no actual need for us to move. We both felt that you and Daniel regarded the house in Stoke as your house with him being the interloper. I guess this was only to be expected as we three had lived there together for five years before we moved to London. I thought that a new house would bring a fresh start. Leroy chose a house near to the school that you and Daniel attended to make it easier for you to get to school and be close to your school friends. It was a bigger house and had a master bedroom with an en-suite bathroom. Daniel, Lilly, and you would all have your own bedrooms, and we made your bedroom the one opposite the bathroom at the other end of the landing from ours so that you could feel a sense of privacy. I think the computer went into the downstairs dining room when we first moved in, but I can't really remember, as everything was about to blow up in another direction not long after we moved.

All my love and affection,

To my very own beautiful daughter,

Mum

xxxx

FIRST INTERLUDE

To My Second Unborn Child

Dear loved one,

You gave me joy for a few months and then left me. What a turbulent family you would have joined! You would have been child number five in a pretty muddled up family with one full sister, one half-sister and two half-brothers. My sister introduced me to the term "blended families" as I did not like the term "stepfamilies" and I feel that this really describes my family, especially if you imagine an electronic blender and picture the blades swirling around as the ingredients are placed in the mixer. You can end up with a great cake, or smoothie or whatever, but the blending involves the breaking down of the individual components, and that is what being in a blended family has felt like to me.

As always, I was totally surprised at the news that I was pregnant. It amazes me that this has been the case each and every time I have conceived. Apart from my first pregnancy, the rest of you have started life against the odds whilst I thought I was taking enough precautions not to conceive! Naturally, I was not taking the ultimate precaution, abstinence from sexual intercourse. Sex is the glue that keeps a marriage together and I was using a lot of glue when you came along!

So although you would have been born into a turbulent family, with toddlers and teens, you were definitely conceived in love and passion and very much wanted. I was taking the contraceptive pill mainly because I had very heavy periods and thought I was too old to cope with another pregnancy or birth. I was really trying to make a go of my job, which was not going well as I had had so much time off following the birth of your sister, Lilly.

Sadly, I was also taking anti-depressants and smoking so that did not give you a good start in life in my womb. Couple this with extreme stress, both at work and at home. For good measure, throw in another car accident with a whiplash injury. Follow that by a fall in the back garden resulting in a trip to accident and emergency on the day that your sister, Sally, and your dad had a massive row in the kitchen. I think it was the fall that did it. It was all just too much for your developing body to cope with, as a couple of weeks afterwards when I started to bleed and ended up in hospital, they told me that you had been dead inside me for a while.

Despite all this, you did give me joy. Both your dad and I were so excited at the news of your arrival. He was overjoyed that Lilly was to have a little brother or sister by me. You would have been our second child together.

I remember clearly the day that I realized you had died. I had been feeling dreadful for a couple of weeks, ever since Sally and your dad had argued so vehemently—the same day that I fell and ended up in hospital and the day that I decided to send Sally to my mum's. So I thought I felt terrible because Sally was at my mum's and I was missing her, and because she had told such lies about your dad that I did not know what to do. I often feel physically sick when I am emotionally sick, so I did not listen to what my body was saying as I thought it was my spirit that was sick. Anyway, your dad and I had gone shopping at Freeport, a shopping center near to where we lived. There was a café upstairs that had a large play area for toddlers and for older children and I was watching Lilly in the toddler play area. Actually I was not watching her; I was crawling around and playing with her because she was reluctant to go in unless I accompanied her. My pants started to feel very wet and I felt very sick. I took her into the toilets and pulled my pants down. To my horror, they were filled with blood, which had small clots in it. I cleaned myself up and put toilet paper in my pants and went back to the play area. I was waiting for your dad who was having a look around the shops whilst I looked after Lilly. In those days, I did not have a mobile phone, so all I could do was wait. It was not very long before your dad returned and as soon as I told him what was happening, he bundled me up and took me home. As soon as we got there, he rang the doctor who advised me to remain lying down and check on the bleeding from time to time. He said that often women do bleed during their pregnancies and the key was to have complete rest. He also advised that if I continued to bleed, your dad should take me to the hospital. Well, I did continue to bleed and ended up in hospital. Over the next twenty-four hours, I was on a roller coaster of emotion: one minute I was hopeful of your survival, the next convinced your life was over.

I lost you. A scan confirmed this.

One of the things that distressed me the most was that one of the staff at the hospital refused to call you a baby or even a fetus; instead she called you fetal waste matter or something like that. They said that because you were under a certain number of weeks old, you did not classify as a fetus. I was fourteen weeks pregnant when this happened and they told me you had died in the womb a couple of weeks earlier, so by my calculations that made you twelve weeks old. I remember lying in the bed weeping with such a huge sense of loss and desolation. I did not know how I was going to carry on, but I did.

Now I believe that you have joined your older sibling in heaven so that makes me feel better, although I often wonder if things would have turned out differently if you had survived. Your departure caused so much grief for your father and me. It was not a grief that was recognized by anyone else; it was an unseen grief because there had been no baby for everyone else to see. Strangers did not know why we were sad, but then again neither did family and friends. Even when people know you have had a miscarriage, they do not understand the grief unless they, too, have been in the same position.

I also want you to know that it was not only me that was grieving your death, but also your father. I was afraid when I lost you because I knew how much he wanted another child. I was afraid that he would go back to drinking in his grief, but he didn't. He was not himself, though. I persuaded him that it was time for Sally to return home. Now more than ever, I wanted her home because I had lost you and I just wanted all my children under one roof. She came back and we started to make plans to move.

One day, I took her and Daniel into the local town where they were meeting friends and came home to spend some time with Lilly and Leroy. Lilly was in the kitchen with your dad, Leroy, when I returned and he was at the sink. Lilly was standing on a stool near him and putting her hands in the water trying to play with the water. I didn't realize it at the time, but he was not coping with the situation or with life. Something snapped and as I walked into the kitchen, he turned the taps on full, filled up the plastic washing up bowl with water and then turned and tipped it all onto the floor. He turned to me and said, "There, she wants to play with water. Now it's easy; it's all over the floor." He left me standing there stunned and went upstairs saying he was going to pack and leave.

I knew that he was angry about something, but I did not know what. I started to clear up the mess in the kitchen. (Yes, I know that I should have made your dad clear up his own mess, but you can't make someone who is packing to leave clear up water from the kitchen floor. If you have a toddler there who might slip and fall, you clear up the water to keep them out of danger.) Obviously, I tried to speak to your dad and begged him not to leave, but he would not speak to me and just brushed past me with a packed bag. Looking back now, I realize that it was another of those *shutdown* situations. There was no row, no shouting, just an ominous silence. He did not even say goodbye, just got in the car and left. That was it.

I was shaking and my whole world came tumbling down around me. I was in a complete and utter state of shock. Here I was thinking that I was just beginning to get my life back in order and this happened. It was so unexpected. He was gone for a week or so and I did not know where he was. I did not hear from him and thought that he had left me for good. I could not eat and I could not sleep. I remember going to pick up Daniel and Sally later that day and telling them that Leroy had left. Lilly was very little so I just tried to reassure her that he had gone away for a while and would be back. I cried a lot, but mostly at night when all the kids were in bed. I continued to look after the kids and go to work, but inside I was a complete wreck. I remember phoning my sponsor from Al Anon. I got a babysitter, and she and I went out to the cinema one evening. She counseled me to just carry on as usual and live one day at a time, one hour, or one minute at a time if need be. So I did and I got through.

Out of the blue, your dad rang me and said that if I wanted him to come back, we would have to move house quickly. Whilst he had been away, he had been to the estate agents and looked at a few houses and had chosen one. He had put an offer in and it had been accepted. Your dad is just like that, hard to explain, hard to live with, impulsive, but deep down he is a good man. I still can't figure him out, but lately, many years later, I have discovered something about him, which explains some of his seemingly erratic behavior. You see, dear child, your dad is on the Autism Spectrum. He has never actually been diagnosed as such, but you now have another brother who is Autistic. Three years after I lost you, and after losing another baby, I had a boy. That boy is called Callum and that boy was diagnosed at age five with Autism. It was when we were learning about ASD (Autism Spectrum Disorder) that your dad recognized himself.

It appears that on that day he walked out on me, he was not actually able to verbalize his feelings. He just tipped over the edge of reasoning. In hindsight, I know that he was experiencing shock and grief over your loss and could not make sense out of losing you. Sally had come back, but the accusations she had made were still rankling in his mind. On the day in question, I had left him alone with Lilly and knowing me, I probably took longer than he was expecting to return to the house. Being Autistic, this is one of the things that he has difficulty dealing with; if someone says they are going to be fifteen minutes and they are in fact sixteen minutes, they are deliberately lying and taking advantage. So on my return, he just flipped and left.

It was not the end of our marriage and we did reconcile, but it shows what grief can do to relationships. Some couples never recover from the loss of a child in whatever circumstances.

One day, baby, I hope to see you in heaven and at least I know that you have been spared some of the pains of this life even if you have missed out on some of the joys.

Goodbye …

Love,

Your Mother

xxxx

LETTER 11

Things Begin to Disintegrate

Dear Daniel,

So why am I writing you these letters? I guess you must know the reason. Even as I sit and type this, I have tears streaming down my face, as there has been so much agony in our lives. What happened to spoil that mother/son relationship between the day you were born to the day I climbed out of a pub toilet window with your sister and left you sitting there fourteen years and ten months later? How could any mother worth her salt accept defeat and get her first born dearly beloved son put into foster care because she could no longer cope with bringing him up? This is the same mother who had felt so abandoned by her own parents, not only as a teenager who was pregnant, but all through her childhood in hostels, children's homes, and boarding schools. How could she abandon her own son? This is the same woman who had it written into her will after your father and I separated, that you, her son, was never to be sent to a boarding school. The thought of you or your sister going through the same feelings of isolation and loneliness that I had felt was so unbearable to me.

It is now nearly ten years since that fateful day and today I am living in Australia whilst you are still in England. All this you know, but what you cannot fully know is what led me to that day in January 2001, which changed the course of both our lives.

The day itself is etched into my brain. Things were not going well in our new "happy" family. Everything looked good on the outside, but really it was rotten to the core, as you know. On the outside, we had just moved to a four-bedroom, detached house. You and Sally were enrolled in a local Secondary School with a fantastic reputation. I had fought to get you enrolled as we had actually lived out of the catchment area when you were first due to be enrolled. Lilly was enrolled at a nursery. Leroy was no longer drinking, was going to AA, and had a good job that he could commute to every day and I was head of department at a Secondary School about thirty minutes away from where we lived. Perfect? Far from it!

My marriage to Leroy was definitely on the rocks. He had left me once already after my first miscarriage, not being able to cope with the grief. You had spent a year in London with your own dad and the whole thing had been disastrous. Sally had only recently returned home from a stint at my mum's, where I sent her for seven weeks. Lilly's eczema was quite severe and she kept me awake most nights with her crying and scratching. I often ended up sleeping on the floor in her room on a quilt with her beside me so that I could rub cream on her in the night to ease her sore skin. I was not coping with my job, mainly due to the fact that I was not getting any sleep and was on a high dose of antidepressants.

It was early 2002 and Christmas had been a nightmare. Before we moved to the house, it had been apparent that you were not yourself at all. You returned from your year at your dad's a very different boy. I noticed a change in your behavior. You started to sleep a lot in the day and were very unresponsive. Your eyes were glazed most of the time. I had had phone calls from school about bizarre behavior, and you were getting in trouble with police quite regularly. I suspected drugs were the cause and it turned out that you had been smoking a lot of cannabis. Actually, I will probably never know the truth about what was going on in your life at this time or what was going on in Leo's life. There were a lot of lies told. All I could see was that you were a very angry, often violent person who would do anything to get money for cannabis or whatever else you were taking. Where had my son gone?

There was a lot of tension in the house. Leroy was at this time what is called in AA circles "a recovering alcoholic." AA and the twelve-step program is deliberately a "selfish" program and the recovering alcoholic is encouraged to put self and sobriety first in every situation. I know the reason for this because once that first drink is taken, they are back on the road to hell on earth for themselves and their families. In order to preserve his sobriety, we had a ban in the house on alcohol. There is also another aspect of AA and that is contained in its name: *anonymity.* Leroy did not want anyone to know either professionally or personally that he was a recovering alcoholic. This of course, led to lies being told on my part to both you and your sister and also to social services, when they eventually got involved. He wanted his anonymity preserved and felt this was essential to his continued sobriety. I was really, really not coping with your aggression, and your anger that was manifesting toward me at every turn. I had decided not to let you have any money because it was apparent to me that any money I gave you, you were using to spend on drugs. We had many conversations about this in which you extolled the virtues of cannabis.

I had lots of advice from people in Al Anon and all of it was that I must be firm and that I must not enable you to continue on your path of drug taking. There were lots of stories told of mothers who had been stabbed and attacked by sons who had a drug problem. I was to be firm and not give in to threats for money. I was to operate a tough love, zero tolerance approach. This I tried and believe me, I was sure it would work. After all, given the choice, what fourteen-year-old would choose cannabis over home and a family?

One day shortly before the fateful day in the pub, we went for a walk. It was snowy, but not snowing. You were angry and accusing me of choosing Leroy over you. I kept telling you that, that was not the issue and that I loved you both. The issue was you had to choose between cannabis and home. I was not going to allow you to take cannabis and continue to live at home. The conversation did not get anywhere. You kept insisting that I was mental; you did not have a problem and all the other mums allowed their teenagers to use cannabis. In fact, they often joined them. What was I to do? This was different. How could I continue? How could I resolve this? I needed help. You needed help.

I would ground you and you would stick your two fingers up at me and go out anyway. Once I threatened that you would lose your room; you did not believe me and went out. Whilst you were out, I moved you out of your room and put you into the smallest room that previously had been Lilly's. Another time, I told you I would lock you out if you went out; you did not believe me and went out. I locked you out. When you came back, I called the police. You had previously told me that the police wouldn't listen to me and would laugh at me. You were right; you acted very sweet in front of them and they did nothing, but told me to ring social services. When I rang social services, they told me that drug taking was a police matter. It was a Catch Twenty-two. We muddled on. Leroy mainly kept out of it in efforts to preserve his sobriety and also being your stepdad he did not want it to come to a situation where you would swear at him and tell him that he was not your real dad. He himself had his own anger management problems and he did not want to get into a confrontational situation with you, as he was scared that his reaction would be extreme. So in reality, although I was married again, I was still a single parent as far as you and Sally were concerned. I, too, had a great fear of being abandoned.

This is not an ideal or healthy way to operate in a so-called blended family and I have often told people that in blended families most of the members of the family feel like they have been through the blender and it is not always a smoothie that comes out! Sometimes, even now, I still feel like we are all actually still going through the blending process and it truly does feel like sharp blades are slicing us up and blending us together.

Back to that fateful day. It was a Sunday. I don't know how much you remember of that day and I know that your memory will not be anything like mine. Up to the point where I left you at the pub, our memories should coincide even if you will only know what you were feeling and I will only know what I was feeling. I only know that it was a day that changed the course of your life and also of mine. It. has taken me a long time to come to terms with this day and even now if I dwell on it for too long, I feel pain in the depths of my being. It has only been years later that I have been able to forgive and feel forgiveness. I still don't really know how or why it ended up as it did or if I could have done anything differently given the circumstances. Only God knows. I spent years going over and over the events of the day and asking myself a lot of what ifs.

Leroy and I had decided to change the carpeted floors in the downstairs of our new home to laminate floors. This was in an effort to ease Lilly's eczema symptoms as we had been told to remove as many carpets as possible. The man who was to do the job had arrived and was unloading all the floorboards off his truck. It was obviously taking its toll and he was struggling. Leroy was helping and he called me and asked me to ask you to give the man a hand. You were lying on the couch in the living room. I asked you to help and you refused. You said, "It's his job. He's getting paid. Why should I help?"

I tried to persuade you, but to no avail. I could see that Leroy was very angry and wanted to avoid a confrontation between you and him, so I asked you to get off the couch and go to your room. You swore at me and refused to move. At this point, I was getting desperate. I hate confrontation so much I just wanted to get you out of there so I could calm you down and talk some sense into you. Why were you being so defiant? Why were you jeopardizing the peace in the house? What would Leroy think? What would he do? I just could not face a confrontation between the two of you, especially not in front of a stranger. Would Leroy turn to drink again as he had in the past to escape the situation? I just had to get you out of the house so we could talk in private. It was Sunday and Leroy and I had an agreement that I needed time alone with you and Sally, without Lilly for a couple of hours at the weekend so I seized this opportunity to say to Leroy that I was taking you both out. That finally got you off the couch; I told you that I was taking you both out for breakfast.

Inside, I was shaking with fear. Outside, I was calm. My body was on autopilot: leave the house, unlock the car, get in the car, seatbelt on, start the car. Sally and you got in the car and I started driving. I actually did not know where I was going to go, as I did not know what would be open in the village at this time on a Sunday morning. The high street was quite deserted—not many people out and about yet, although it was late morning. Most of the shops were closed, as were the cafés. At the end of the high street, there is a little café that was open. I stopped and parked feeling relieved that at least I had found somewhere we could eat. Maybe after you had eaten, we could talk like human beings.

Things did not go well in the café. From the moment you entered, you started to complain. You didn't want to eat there; the food was crap. We sat down, you very reluctantly, and the waitress gave us a couple of menus. They were serving breakfast food and I knew that you love this type of food, so I made a few suggestions. Sally chose some food, and so did I. All the while, your complaining was getting louder and louder. You pushed the menu away and insisted that you would not eat anything. You swore at me, calling me obscene names, shouting general obscenities in the air, about the owner and the food. You shouted that the owner was a pig and that the place and the food were disgusting and filthy.

I said, "Okay, you don't have to eat here, but Sally and I are hungry so we will eat."

You got louder and louder, swearing and complaining. The café is very, very small, with only three small tables in the section where we were and the other customers were obviously becoming uncomfortable with the situation. Sally insisted that she was hungry and told you to shut up, but you were not listening. Finally, I could take it no more and got up and left, never to return to that particular café. Your verbal abuse continued as we left and got into the car. By this time, I was actually terrified; your whole manner was very aggressive. I had nowhere to go; I certainly couldn't go home as you were still ranting. I was trying hard to remain calm, but felt like my whole world was falling apart. This was my son, my only son, whom I love more than words could ever say and I was petrified of him. I really, really wanted you to stop shouting and swearing. I really, really wanted you to stop and just say, "Sorry, Mum."

I just wanted you to stop swearing and calling me names and listen to me. Instead, you demanded that we go to a pub, as you were sure that they would be open. I did not want to go to a pub because pubs are part of the problem. They serve alcohol and alcohol is a problem in our family. Your dad is a drinking alcoholic, you seem to have a drinking problem, and Leroy is a recovering alcoholic. I certainly wanted to be as far away as possible from a venue that serves alcohol. Alcohol never improves a situation; it always, always makes things worse. I was scared of being in a pub with you.

We drove around. There was literally nowhere else open in the village, so I drove to a pub just out of town, which is more of a family pub and serves meals. By this time, it was nearly midday and we discovered that the pub was due to open at midday. We waited until it opened and went in. You seemed a little happier, but soon it all started again. You asked me to order you a beer as you were fourteen and pubs are allowed to serve alcohol to fourteen-year-olds as long as they are having a meal. I refused and this caused another outburst. You swore at me again and accused me of being a hypocrite. You reminded me that on a previous occasion I had bought you a drink, so what was different about today? Out came a long spiel about me being abnormal and over-sensitive to alcohol—just because your dad is an alcoholic, doesn't make you one—just because you want one drink, doesn't mean you are going to get drunk. I stood my ground and we ordered some food.

Drinks had to be ordered separately and bought at the bar. Sally was thirsty and asked for a drink. I was hemmed in by you at a table; you blocked my way to the bar to get the drinks and held my arm strongly, trying to get through to me what a useless piece of crap I was and a useless mother. I decided to send Sally to the bar to get the soft drinks and got some money out of my purse to give to her. Your eyes lit up and you offered to go. Of course, I insisted that Sally go to the bar. You knew it was because I did not trust you with the money and this inflamed you even further. If it was bad before, it got worse. You were really on a roll and just couldn't seem to stop. I asked you to stop and your laughing reply was, "Make me."

At this point, I wanted to die, literally die. My life did not seem worth living. I had no answers. I had nothing to call upon, no human experience to let me see how to cope with this conflict and this anger. I knew I must not give in as I had in the past. Maybe if I had trusted you with the money on that occasion and you had returned to the table with the soft drinks and handed me the change, everything would have been different.

Maybe not.

We will never know.

I had reached a point of utter desperation. I needed to go home as we had now been out for a few hours. Leroy would be expecting me and Lilly would miss me, but I couldn't leave, as you were still angry. I was scared that if I went home and took you with me, there would be an almighty row in the house between you and Leroy and that one or both of you would get hurt. You were just so angry that I did not know what to do. This was like never before. I just could not communicate with you, and I couldn't get through to you the seriousness of the situation. I couldn't make you understand that something had to change and that I couldn't cope. You were taunting me as I again brought up the subject of cannabis and alcohol and again stated that I was not going to allow them in the house and that you were going to have to abide by the rules of the house. You continued to taunt me, to insist that I couldn't make you do anything you didn't want to do. I mentioned the police and you again reminded me that they would just laugh at me. I talked about social services and you said they would just laugh at me and tell me to get on with it. Social services are there to protect children from bad parents not to help parents deal with normal teenage sons like you!

We talked about the situation that very morning and you couldn't acknowledge that your behavior was in any way out of order. As far as you were concerned, it was your house, you could lie on the couch as long as you liked, speak how you liked and you should not have been asked to help a tradesman who was getting paid for his work. I did kind of understand what you were saying about the tradesman, but the situation was not really like that. It was just a way of being polite and joining in with a venture that was to improve our living conditions. It would maybe have involved five minutes of your time and shown good will and showed that you respected me, but you couldn't see this because you do not respect me at all. I repeated that I would have to turn to social services if I couldn't get through to you. You laughed loudly and continued to swear at me; your every posture was mocking and threatening.

As I write this letter, I am reliving the day and tears are welling up in my eyes. I have to keep stopping and composing myself so that I can continue.

After Sally came back with the drinks, things carried on in the same vein; she was not silent during this time and joined the conversation from time to time. She was trying to persuade you to cooperate, but you also had a go at her a few times.

Do you remember that you and she had always fought with each other and were extremely jealous of my affection? At bedtimes when you were little, you both used to time the amount of time I spent with the other and I had to make sure I alternated between the two of you having the final goodnight.

You would not listen to me and you would not listen to her.

I sat in the pub and felt utterly hopeless, useless and scared. Nothing I said seemed to be getting through to you. This boy that I loved beyond measure was sitting next to me spewing vile contempt at me and at everything that I said. You were even trapping me in my seat so I could not move away. Finally, you needed to go to the toilet and I just wanted to run, so as soon as you disappeared behind the toilet door, I grabbed Sally and said, "Come quickly, we have to get out of here before Daniel comes back from the toilet."

We ran to the car, but we were not quick enough. You saw us through the pub window and came running out after us. As I tried to get into the car, you grabbed my arm and started swearing at me again, pulling me away from the car door. There was no way I could return home with you in the state you were in and I was now petrified of what you might do to me or to Sally.

We returned to the pub and sat down. The conversation continued on in the same vein with you now laughing at me for trying to run away and leave you there. There was no respite; honestly, Daniel, I thought that my world was ending, I kept thinking that I had to go on for the sake of Sally and Lilly, but at that moment, I would quite happily have ended my own life. I could not see any point in carrying on living if this is what it was all about. My own son hated me and loved alcohol and cannabis more than me. He wanted those things more than he wanted to please me or be part of our family. My own son despised me. I was scared of my own son. Was this the son that had grown from the baby that had changed my life nearly fifteen years before? Was this the boy that was joint top goal scorer for his year eight football team, was in the lawn tennis association, was chosen for gym squad at eight years old, was a great cross-country runner and who seemed to be good at everything he touched? Was this the boy whom teachers told me could easily get 10 Grade A, GCSEs when he entered secondary school? Was this the same boy who slept in my bedroom for eighteen months after his granddad died? Was this the same boy who used to sit on my lap sucking his thumb and twiddling my hair until he was eight? Was this the same boy who had said to me in a very frightened voice that he would eat s—- to come back and live with me during the year he lived with his dad? It was the same boy on the outside, but I knew that it was not the same boy on the inside; that boy had disappeared. It was like watching a TV program with the sound turned off. I could see your angry face. I could see your mouth opening and closing. I could see the look of scorn in your eyes, but I could not see my boy anywhere.

It really was the proverbial straw that broke the camel's back. I knew that my marriage to Leroy was also on the point of breaking down as he was not coping well with the reality of life since he had stopped drinking. Drinking had been his escape from reality and without that crutch, he had to face the stress and strains of normal family life—only our family life was not really normal. I thought about Lilly and about her having to go through what you and Sally had been through with the breakup of my marriage to your father. What would happen to her and to Sally if I took you back home? Something had to give, to change. I just knew I could not continue to manage to look after Sally and Lilly, work full time, and deal with what you were going through.

(I did not know that I was actually on the point of a mental breakdown that would eventually see me walk out of my teaching job one day never to return. This breakdown would eventually lead me to turn to the God of my youth and bring hope to our seemingly hopeless situation.)

I formed a plan. I would get Sally and myself to the toilets and see if I could escape from there. Honestly, Daniel, at that time and in those circumstances, I did not feel that I had any other option open to me, but to remove Sally and myself from the pub, leaving you there. We managed to get away from you and went to the toilet. There was a low window in there and we managed to get it open. I don't really know how

Sally felt at this time, but she was just as eager as I was to escape. We climbed through the window, ran to the car, jumped in, and I drove off as fast as I could. I was sobbing and shaking all the way home. When I got home, I felt immense relief, but not for long as the reality of what I had done sank in. At least at home, I had time to think and try to figure out what to do. I was totally stunned at the way the day had turned out.

When I first left the house, I had visions of coming home with two happy smiling teenagers, well fed and with all grievances aired and if not settled at least on the way to settlement. You would walk back into the house all apologetic for the behavior you had displayed prior to going out, and for the moment at least, the crisis would be averted. We would all live to tell another tale. This, of course, had not happened; the crisis was in fact here. I remember people in Al Anon sharing that every crisis is an opportunity for change. I must take this opportunity. I must not try to avoid this crisis. I must face it head on. Things could not continue in the same way. I must be firm, or risk losing everything; I was so scared of losing Leroy, failing at a second marriage, having to bring up Lilly as a single parent, and not being able to handle you in the home. I was scared that if I weakened, we would all be in danger. When you got angry, Daniel, you were scary; it seemed there was nothing that would stop you. It seemed that using cannabis had changed you. I felt I had always been able to get through to you before you started using it, but not anymore. Okay, you still got angry when things did not go your way and you had always been very lively and argumentative, but in the end, love had won out and you had eventually seemed to comply.

As you were growing up, people had suggested to me that you were what they called *hyperactive*. A few had even told me that I should get you put on Ritalin, but I resisted, and anyway I do not believe that it would have been a good thing to do. Knowing what I know now about food and how the additives and colors and preservatives affect children, I should have given you better food choices when you were growing up, but at the time, I thought I was feeding you good food. I found out early on that if you had a drink of cola you would literally climb the walls afterwards and be totally uncontrollable, so I limited the cola that you drank, much to your disgust! As a substitute, I would buy caffeine-free, diet Coke, which I now believe was probably worse for you in that it contains aspartame or similar sugar substitutes. Having said all this, I did my best with the knowledge that I had at the time. I loved you and I thought that this was enough to get me through. I had no personal experiences of normal family life as a teenager. I had no brothers so didn't really know or understand how teenage boys thought or acted. I had no boyfriends until the age of seventeen and that boyfriend was twenty-two. My own father was not a stereotypical alpha male: he had been a conscientious objector in World War II and had no interest whatsoever in sport; he was very strict and he played the piano when he was angry or upset. It was absolutely impossible to argue with him even if you wanted to because he refused to argue or debate anything. What he said was law. Period!

Anyway, back to the day that changed the course of both our lives in unimaginable ways. Naturally, you discovered that Sarah and I had left the pub. Not long after I got home, I received a phone call from a member of the staff at the pub who asked me to come and pick you up. She said that she was going to have to call the police if I did not come. I told her that I was not coming and that she should call the police if she felt she needed to. Even at this point, the day could have turned out differently; although the pub was a couple of miles from where we lived, it was still not too far to walk. If on that day you had decided to walk home and on that walk had thought things through and in effect walked off your anger and appeared contrite at the door, things may have taken a different turn of events. We may have been able to carry on as before and even come through the crisis unscathed. Again, this did not happen and actually I do not believe that things would have turned out any differently in the end. The only way things would have turned out differently would have been if you had not been involved in taking drugs at that time. Once drugs enter the situation, nothing proceeds as normal. In fact, there is no normal. There is no reasoning. There is only drugs: taking them, wanting them, stealing for them, being bad tempered without them. Relationships do not matter; the only thing that matters is getting the money to buy the drugs, somehow, anyhow. There would have come a time when you would have had to leave home.

I know that even now you do not accept that drugs were the main issue here, but from where I am standing, that is the only explanation I can give for the way in which you changed. Every conversation with you at the time revolved around cannabis; you took every opportunity to try to persuade me that I should allow you to take it and allow you money for it. You were obsessed with it. Taking it was more important to you than maintaining or restoring family relationships and it continued to be the same for the next few years. It is possible that this particular day could have ended differently, but there would have come a day when our paths diverged. You always maintained that I was extra sensitive about drugs and alcohol because of my experiences with your own father and also because of my experiences with Leroy and this is true. It opened my eyes to the world of alcoholism and addiction, and I was determined that I was not going to enable my own son to become trapped in this world. If you got trapped, it would be your own doing. I was not going to help you in any way.

The outcome of leaving you in the pub was that the landlady called the police who then called me. They said they had you with them and could they bring you home. I told them what had happened in the pub and said that I was scared of you and did not want you home. It had finally come to this. Amazingly, they did not laugh at me as you had said they would. They got in touch with social services and found you a place in temporary foster care. They brought you round so I could get some clothes together for you to take with you. By this time, I think the reality of what was happening was sinking in with you, and yes, this time you started to cry and begged me to let you come back home. Everything in me wanted to just take you in my arms and gather you to myself, but I knew that I could not do this, as I did not believe that anything would have changed. You would still be trying to get money to get cannabis, you would still be defying me at every turn, and you would now also hold me accountable for leaving you in the pub.

With great sorrow, I saw you drive away in the police van. Really, my life felt as if it had ended and my self-respect definitely left on that day. I was a completely useless mother who had to give her beloved son up to foster care. So although I had all the grand thoughts of being strong and not being the one to enable my son to kill himself by using drugs, it didn't help me at all at that time. I still felt like the lowest of the low. How could I live with myself? I was a complete and utter failure; there was nothing worth continuing for. The person who had survived boarding school, bullying, sexual assault, forced abortion, abandonment, an alcoholic marriage, held at gunpoint, physical assault, sexual betrayal through adultery, an alcoholic marriage, post-natal depression, a messy divorce, death of my father and a close friend in a couple of months, being a single mother and building a successful career, being in debt, another alcoholic marriage, another dose of post-natal depression, and a miscarriage was not surviving this. This was not happening to me; I was doing it.

Daniel, only you will know what you were thinking and feeling on that day, or even if you can remember it clearly. I remember that when we met two years ago and had the day together, we went through all the things that have happened since that day that you asked me to fill you in on some of the details and order of events because you said that your memory of the time was hazy. One of the things you wanted me to clarify was whether Leroy and I had become Christians and then kicked you out or if we had kicked you out and then become Christians. I was able to assure you that at the time we kicked you out, we were far from being Christians. We were living without hope and it was only when we became Christians that the possibility of you returning home became a reality.

So why am I telling you all this now? Am I trying to absolve myself; am I trying to show you how bad you were and how good I was? Not at all! My reason for writing this letter is to tell you once and for all that I love you. I always have and I always will. I want to you to know that above all else. What we lost those years was trust. I did not trust you. It is a popular misconception that love is enough in these situations, but where there is substance abuse, be it alcohol or drugs or any other intoxicating addiction, love is not enough. Wisdom, trust, and recovery are needed along with a large dose of perseverance.

As ever,

Mum

xxxx

LETTER 12

The Yoyo Years Commence

Dear Daniel,

What followed that fateful day when I left you in the pub was, for me, a complete nervous breakdown. If I had thought that putting you in the hands of social services would be the thing that would ease the strain on the rest of the family and also bring you quickly to your senses, I was wrong. Because Leroy was a member of AA, which is by nature anonymous and because he was not long into his recovery, he was very sensitive about anyone knowing that he was a recovering alcoholic, particularly any official authorities He did not want it on record anywhere. So as a result of this, he was very angry with me that it had been mentioned during my initial meetings with social services. He felt that it was irrelevant and not the business of either the police or social services. This put a real strain on our marriage at the time, as he felt that I had betrayed his anonymity. It also meant that I had to back-track on some of the things that I had said in consultation with social services. This in turn, I felt, made me look unreasonable. In discussions about your return, one of the stipulations I made was that there was to be no alcohol or drugs in your body or on your person. Many a time you mocked and laughed at me for this stance, but I also felt that social services thought that this stance was severe for a fourteen-year-old boy. I, of course, could not bring up one of the reasons for this was alcohol-ism in the home.

Your dad came up to see you on the day after I left you in the pub. There was a meeting between our family and social services and he offered to have you back to live with him, but you refused that option. You ended up going to live with a foster family in a town about ten miles away. It was arranged that I would visit with you twice a week. Initially, I asked for supervised visits because I was actually very afraid of what you would say and do to me, but after a couple of weeks, I would pick you up and take you out for a couple of hours.

There was a bit of relief at home outwardly as there was not the con-stant tension in the home of an angry, defiant boy, whose one goal seemed to be to get money. But do you know what, Daniel? You were a constant presence with me. I can honestly say that I never stopped thinking about you, wondering where you were, what you were doing, how you were coping. I had enormous feelings of failure. As you know,

I was a teacher all the time that you were growing up and when this happened, I was Head of Department at a Secondary School. One of the subjects that I taught was called PSE (Personal, Social, Education). This involved tackling many topics including relationships and the use of alcohol and drugs. I was the kind of teacher that many of the pupils I taught spoke to about very personal issues. I counseled them on relationships with their parents, using drugs, underage sex, and the like. So here I was at school, spending time with other parents' children and listening to their problems and trying to help them whilst in my own life, everything was in a shambles. My own son in foster care! This could not be right; what a fraud I was! What a complete and utter failure I was as a parent, indeed even as a person. What a mess I had made of my life. I did not want to carry on living. I was just going through the motions.

One Saturday in March 2001, I left the house completely distraught. Leroy and I had argued and he had smashed my mobile phone. I was completely desolate and ready for divorce and or death. I had already walked out of my job one day before the end-of-school bell and had not returned, not even to pick up my belongings. The doctor had put me on anti-depressants and I was seeing a psychologist and a counselor. I was not sleeping at night, partially through worry about you and partially because of Lilly's eczema which was so severe at that time that I was spending most of the night in with her, creaming her legs and body and trying to stop her from scratching and crying. I was completely ready to give up and could see no solutions to any of the difficult situations in my life. All my pride had vanished. Lilly was in her pushchair and I was walking down the street in the small town where we lived. I remembered a leaflet that had come through the door advertising some special services in local churches. I was not sure why, but I crossed the road and looked at the door of one of the local churches that was attached to a bookshop. My mother had taken me to the café and bookshop a couple of times when she had been visiting and I knew that it was a Pentecostal church because I had been brought up in that denomination. I noted the time of the service the following day. I then went into a mobile phone shop and looked at prices for a new mobile phone and decided to risk walking home although I was not sure if Leroy would still be angry when I got home.

I guess the necessities of life prevailed on that day. I had to look after Lilly; who would look after her if I left? I had to look after Sally; who would look after her if I left? When I got home, Leroy was very quiet.

He told me to look for a new phone if I wanted, so I took that as some sort of apology although he never said sorry. We carried on as normal. Later that night whilst creaming Lilly, I thought again about the church. I decided that the following day, I was going to go to the church and as I lay there on the floor with Lilly beside me on the thick quilt that I had laid down beside her little bed, I prayed and I told God what a mess I had made of my life and I asked him to forgive me. I knew that the Bible taught that Jesus had died for me and that he had risen again and that because of this, I could be reconciled to God. Really, it was not complicated. I just accepted that Jesus was who he was, accepted that his death on the cross and resurrection three days later had somehow made amends for my sin and entrusted my life to him. When I think about it now, I would say that it was at that point that I remembered my Creator. I realized that there was *a power greater than I* as they say in the twelve steps of Al-Anon and that that power was the God of the Bible. I had a great sense of God's love for me and knew that he cared for me and I relinquished my life to him.

The next morning, I got up as usual and got Lilly her breakfast keeping a close eye on the time. Leroy was up and just before I was about to leave for church, I told him where I was going and asked him to come along with us. I think I showed him the leaflet that had come through the door. I really did not know what to expect, but I had decided to go whether or not he came, too, and whatever his reaction might be. Maybe he sensed I was serious, maybe not; whatever the reason, he said something like, okay, let's go, and we all got in the car. Later, he told me that what he really thought of doing was swearing at me, but when the words came out he was agreeing to come along.

When we got to the church, we sat on the back row with Lilly in her pushchair in the aisle. I don't remember much of the service except that I somehow felt I had come home. There was a visiting speaker from the mission that was in town and he basically explained who Jesus was and what Jesus had done. I can't really remember his exact words. At the end, he prayed and he asked if there was anyone in the service who would like to accept Jesus. He said that if there was, the person should put up their hand so that he could see it and so that someone could talk to them afterwards. I had my eyes closed, but heard the preacher say that someone had put their hand up. After the prayer, I turned to Leroy and was amazed to see that he was crying. It turned out that it was he who had put his hand up. Now that truly did amaze me! The rest is history; in the same weekend, Leroy and I both became Christians quite independently of each other. It was amazing because it also seemed like there had been an invisible barrier between us and that barrier came down on that morning.

To anyone who is not a Christian, this probably sounds really weird and stupid and I guess that is what it must have seemed like to you. What it meant in reality for you was that there was now a real chance of you coming back home. You see, when you are a Christian, you are forgiven by God, but it does not stop there; you, then, have an obligation to forgive others. This meant that we needed to forgive you and keep on forgiving you whatever the circumstances. Leroy had been very resistant to you coming back on home visits, but after this, we agreed to home visits and started making negotiations with social services for you to come back on overnight/weekend visits with a view to you coming back home to live. I remember telling you that we had become Christians and that we wanted to work at trying to get you back to live at home, but that it was up to you to prove that you could be drug free.

There then followed a series of home visits, which resulted in it being agreed that you would come back and live with us at the end of the school year at the beginning of August. That would make a total of seven months that you were in foster care. You were now fifteen and I was just hoping against hope that I could at least keep you on the straight and narrow until you were sixteen and had finished school. We basically only had one rule: there was to be no alcohol or drugs in your body or on your person at home. You agreed.

You had been expelled from the school you were attending whilst you were in foster care and Leroy and I appealed the decision and went to a panel meeting to argue your case. We explained that we had now become Christians and also that you had been spending more time back at home and were coming back to live with us. We said that we felt you would make a real effort to do well at school and obey the rules and that you really wanted to make a success of being back at home and returning to school. We also made the case that moving you to another school in Year Eleven would be detrimental to you achieving any success at GCSE Level as you were halfway through courses and would probably not be able to follow the same courses in another school.

We lost the appeal and your expulsion was upheld. At the time, I thought it was very unfair, but there was nothing more that Leroy or I could do. It took a while for the powers that be to find you another school and for that time, I was ordered to keep you away from the school premises during school hours. I don't know if you remember, but I tried to get you to do schoolwork at home, but not much got done and you were always chomping at the bit to get down to school when it finished for the day so that you could meet up with your friends.

It was just after we were reunited that I had my second miscarriage whilst we were visiting Nana in Wales. In September, Leroy, Sally, Lilly, you, and I went for a week's holiday. Leroy was actually on a mission trip and was sleeping in local churches whilst we were booked into a caravan park. I wanted to go to as many of the mission events as possible, but you were not keen so I agreed to let you stay in the caravan by yourself. This was a mistake as when I returned, the caravan smelled of aftershave and I could see evidence of *bong* making in the bin. This was a sure sign that you had some dope and that you had been smoking it. You, of course, denied it and told me a tale about how it was the new way to smoke cigarettes! (I was still smoking at this time and one of the agreements we had had on your return home was that you would be allowed to smoke cigarettes.) After that, I would not leave you alone in the caravan and forced you to come with me to some of the crusade meetings.

The week was filled with incidents; on one occasion, you tore off one of the caravan doors to get to Sally after an argument and believe me I was close to giving up the holiday. Lilly's skin became infected and she had open sores all over her torso. I somehow managed to hold it all together and get Lilly to the hospital. We also managed to go to B and Q to get some hinges and tools and fixed the caravan door.

The week also had some happy memories and I have two pictures, which I keep in my Bible, that show you, Sally, and Lilly sitting on a bench with the sea behind and you, Sally, and Lilly sitting on three swings. In the second picture, Lilly is in the middle and you are all holding hands. They are some of the sweetest pictures that I have.

At this point, although I knew it was going to be tough, I thought there was hope that we could make it as a family and that you were back for good, but this was not to be.

After the holiday, we returned home and things seemed to disintegrate quite quickly. On September 10, 2001 you wanted to go out in the town and I told you to stay in. The school had rung me and complained that you had been harassing some of the women teachers on the street so as a consequence, I wanted you to stay in; basically, I grounded you for the night. You were not having a bar of it, so completely defied me and went out, sticking two fingers up at me as you went. This time I decided I was going to go out and find you. Sally seemed to think that there was going to be a big fight in the town and she was sure that you would be part of it. Leroy could not come with me because of Lilly, so I rang the pastor of our church and he agreed to help me look for you on the streets. Another woman from the church also came along. After about an hour of looking, we finally found you, standing, drinking, in the middle of some local youths with a six-pack in one hand and an open beer in the other, which you were happily throwing down your neck. Of course, after getting you into the car I now had another dilemma; we could not go home because you had alcohol in your body. After ringing around, it was agreed that you would go and stay at another church member's house for the night and we would decide what to do in the morning.

In the morning, I picked you up and took you home. I grounded you to your room and Leroy and I discussed what we should do. We did not want to kick you out again, but it was clear that you were not abiding by the rule. We decided that we would ground you to your room for a week and hoped that this would deter you from repeating the behavior. Soon you started shouting out, "Mum, Mum, come and look at this. Leroy, Leroy, they are bombing America." Of course, it was the 9/11 bombing of the Twin Towers in New York and it was live footage on TV. We were so shocked that we allowed you out of your room and we all sat and watched the event and the aftermath on the TV downstairs. So you could say that world events had a play in your diminished punishment that day. Sadly, you continued to break our no-drugs-or-alcohol rule and I was finding it increasingly hard to keep you under control. I was due to have an eye operation in November and asked social services if I could have two weeks respite care for you whilst I recovered. We had a meeting at the house and you requested to go and live with a friend of yours in town, whose mother was a foster parent. I refused permission because I had heard that the mother was a known drug dealer, but you got social services to ring your dad and he gave permission for you to go there for the two weeks. Of course, you shouted and screamed at me and denied that the woman was a drug dealer and you told me I was insane. My hands were tied. There seemed to be nothing I could do once your dad had given permission. It just goes to show that the law is an ass, because as you have now admitted, there were a lot of drugs in that house and so, living there, you progressed deeper and deeper into the world of drugs and crime.

After that stay, you did not really want to come back home to live. Another school was found for you in Crewe and you started to attend there. It was not long before I received a phone call to say that you had been permanently suspended from that school, too. The Head of Year who rang me said that you were the scariest pupil he had had the occasion to meet in all his twenty-two years of teaching experience. No provision was made for your schooling from that point on because they did not formally expel you; they just put you on indefinite suspension, so technically you still had a school. You were in Year Eleven and the powers that be were just biding time until your sixteenth birthday. I understood why they did not want you in school, but again, I thought it was unfair and thought that they should have expelled you, so that you then could have access to home tutors.

After Christmas, which you came home for, you said that you wanted to go back and live at your mate's house. We could not force you to stay at home because we knew that you did not want to be there and you did not like our rules. We had failed miserably in trying to keep you away from drugs and alcohol and I knew that they were more important to you than living at home. There were a few occasions over these years that you said that I had chosen Leroy above you. Each time, I remember saying that in fact you had chosen drugs and alcohol over living at home with me. It is true that other parents may have been able to deal with the situation better than I did; it is true that other parents would have allowed you to stay at home and use drugs. Someone asked me the other day whether I thought I did the right thing when I kicked you out initially. My response was I am not sure if it was the right thing or the wrong thing; it is just what I did. I know my motives were to show you that I was serious about the whole drug and alcohol thing and also were an attempt to keep the rest of the family together. You see having been married to two alcoholics, I just was not prepared to go through it all again and that is where I thought we were headed. The fact that you would not obey that rule, or any other rule for that matter, if it did not suit you, meant that I found it impossible to parent you.

Still I loved you and longed for you to be at home with me. We booked a holiday in Canada and in faith, invited you to come along with us. I was so happy that you wanted to come and was really praying that the break from your friends would help to break the cycle you were in. The trip itself was a good one. There was still some, bad feeling between us, but we had a good holiday and you seemed to be a little like your old self. Canada was always a good place for us and I really enjoyed being with my sister and her husband. You got on well with your two cousins and generally everything went well. One day you asked me if I would ask my sister if you could stay in Canada for a while when we returned because you did not want to go back to your old life. She and her husband agreed and it was a very happy and hopeful time.

We returned home and I was so excited. By this time, your room had become an office, so I set about making the garage into a new bedroom for you. The plan was that you would return home, sit your GCSEs and then, having proved you could stay off drugs and alcohol for a few months, we would apply for you to return to Canada to live with my sister and attend school or college there.

All seemed to be going well. I was beginning to get excited and felt happy for the first time in many years.

Love,

Mum

xxxx

LETTER 13

In the Meantime...

Dear Sally,

As you know, after we moved nearer to your secondary school, all hell broke loose in our house with your brother Daniel. Of course, whilst all this stuff was going on with Daniel, you were living your own life and as it turns out, it was not very pretty either. I look back now and realize that I was obsessed with trying to sort out the situation with Daniel and often just assumed that everything was okay with you. As always, I felt I was doing the best I could in a difficult situation. Little did I know! I have often tried to juggle balls and have never succeeded, not even with two balls. In life, it appears I have much the same capabilities, i.e., I keep dropping the ball, and at times have not really been able to juggle all the competing roles in my life successfully.

With you, things seemed to be calm after your return from your Nana's. She had taken you to church whilst you were there and you had decided to become a Christian. Although I was not a Christian, I was happy about your decision. I hoped that it would give you peace and some direction in life. All through your life, you had asked me to pray with you and at times you were very worried that I did not believe in God.

All I can say about the Daniel situation is that it seems that not only was I suffering from some kind of depression, but also great grief. I could not understand why Daniel had seemed to choose drugs over family. My focus was to get him off drugs and back living at home.

You, on the other hand, seemed to be doing fine. You were back at the same school and had reconnected with all your friends. After all, you had only been away for seven weeks. You did not seem to be unduly upset about me kicking Daniel out; in fact, you often fought with him and seemed relieved that he was not at home. I gave you a belated thirteenth birthday party as you had been at Nana's when you turned thirteen. It was a bit of a disaster as even though I was in the house with Lilly, you and your friends turned off all the lights downstairs and got up to a bit of nonsense. To this day, I am not sure exactly what was going on, but I remember turning on all the lights and screaming at you all. I made you all sit in lines in the sitting room whilst your friends waited for their parents to pick them up. I made a mental note—no more parties for teenagers in my house! The reality was so different from my expectation of always having a houseful of happy teenagers, listening to music, chatting, and playing board or card games whilst drinking tea and cool drinks. So even as an adult, it seems I was still very naïve in some respects.

You were allowed to go out with friends often, and you did. I trusted you. After Leroy and I became Christians, you came along to church with us and got involved in a youth group there. You came on holiday with us to the Lake District and visited Scotland and Wales with us. You seemed to be doing well at school and I thought that you were very conscientious. Of course, there were a lot of things going on that I knew nothing about. Daniel would tell me that you were often up to no good and I would confront you and you would deny it and I would believe you. I thought that he was just trying to get you into trouble and to justify his own way of life.

I made special time with you every week, and once a week, I would take you out on your own. We usually ended up going to a local shopping center and I would stand outside changing cubicles in cheap fashion shops for what seemed like hours, whilst you tried on clothes. It was a frustrating time for both of us as you were angry if I hurried you and I was upset if you made me stand outside too long. There were invariably heated discussions about items of clothing that you wanted that either I could not afford or did not approve of. So it goes with teenage daughters and their middle-age mothers.

In some ways, I guess I have not been a typical mother in that I am not really interested in makeup, fashion, jewelry accessories, or any of that girly stuff. I am a get up and go person, who rarely even blow-dries my hair. I do wear make up from time to time and I do like nice clothes, but it is not my passion. I like to claim that I am too busy to apply makeup every day, but in reality, I did not use it much as a teenager and we all know that teenagers have all the time in the world! Actually, I was not allowed to wear it as a young teenager as my dad thought it was straight from the pits of hell, but that is a different story. I wasn't allowed to wear trousers or jeans either, but I love wearing them now.

What I am really trying to say is that I knew it was important to make time for you and you alone and I did, but the time did not always turn out to be as fun as I always imagined it would be. I could see that you were growing into a stunningly beautiful girl; in fact, your face was so beautiful that I did not understand why you needed to apply so much makeup and so often, but there we go. You dated a few boys, but I never really saw any of them. There were no longstanding boyfriends that I knew about. You talked about your friends a lot and often told me that they were the most important people in your life.

I will never forget May 22, 2001, as it was the day that the baby I lost whilst you were in Wales was due and I approached the day with sadness and with regret about what might have been. Social services scheduled a meeting with me on that day to discuss Daniel's progress in foster care and to start making arrangements for him to return home. Whilst I was in the meeting, I had a phone call from your school. You had broken a collarbone whilst demonstrating a hurdle jump to the class in P.E. and I was to go straight to the hospital. What a day! I had to leave the meeting and rush to the hospital.

It was quite a bad break and of course, being your collarbone could not be put into plaster. You were given a sling and some painkillers and sent on your way. It really put you out of action for a couple of months—story of your life. For the first few weeks, you could not even dress yourself or have a wash without help. I even had to help you going to the toilet for the first few days. It must have been very embarrassing for you and extremely painful, but not for me. After all, you were and are still my baby. At least it took my mind off the baby that I lost for a while.

Love,

Mum

xxxx

SECOND INTERLUDE

To My Third Unborn Child

Dear loved one,

Your death surprised me the most out of my three unborn children. You would have been the fifth child in a "blended" family with two older sisters and two older brothers. Your death came on the day before your dad was due to be baptized, during the first week that your brother Daniel had come back to live with us. Go figure!

After my first miscarriage, I stopped taking contraceptive pills. I continued to smoke and I continued to take anti-depressants, but I knew it was possible for me to conceive and I knew that your dad desperately wanted more children. The miscarriage, along with other things that were going on in my life, caused me to have a breakdown. I walked out of my job in the February following the miscarriage, and one month after kicking out your older brother Daniel for taking drugs. I was receiving counseling, seeing an occupational therapist, attending stress management classes, and applying for early retirement from teaching on the advice of my union and my psychiatrist. I knew how grieved your dad had been after my miscarriage and deep down I must have thought that having another baby would heal that grief and make things better between us. Of course, anyone with half a brain knows that having a baby does not heal a relationship; if the relationship is not good, it is more likely to break it. Children only strengthen a good marriage (although I do realize that many childless couples have great marriages.)

So you were really my only planned baby. It is a disputable honor! I was once again overjoyed to discover I was pregnant. This time even more so as I was not working, your dad and I had become Christians, we were trying to get Daniel to agree to stop taking drugs to enable him to come back home, and I felt that God was blessing me with another baby.

When I became a Christian, I made a decision to be more "open" and accepting of other Christians. Some of the Christians at the church we had started to attend knew our circumstances and knew that we had recently lost a baby. A few of them believed that basically if you asked God for something and believed he would give it to you, then he was obliged to do so. It didn't seem quite right to me, but not wishing to return to the cynical person that I had been for so many years, I decided to give it a go. I actually prayed and told God we wanted another baby, but I asked that I would not get pregnant again if it was going to end in a miscarriage. So as a result, when I found out that I was pregnant again, I was over the moon. I thought I was untouchable and that nothing would go wrong; after all, we had prayed in faith, believing God would answer our prayers, and here I was pregnant again. God would not allow me to get pregnant if something was going to go wrong.

So when I started to bleed, my heart sank. How could this be? What about my faith that everything would be okay this time? What was happening? I couldn't be losing my baby.

I was at my mum's house in Wales with your dad and Daniel, Sally, and Lilly. It was Thursday. We were all there for a week's holiday and your dad was going to get baptized in the sea on the Saturday. Daniel was finally back as part of the family and all our church friends were coming down for the day to watch your dad get baptized. I told your dad that I needed to have a rest and I hoped that by lying down the bleeding would stop, but it didn't. Finally, after a couple of hours, I had to break the news to your dad that I needed to go to hospital. He was distraught.

When we arrived at hospital, they admitted me straight away and put me on a maternity ward. At this point, the medical staff was not sure whether or not I would lose you. I kept losing blood, but they kept saying that my blood tests showed I was still pregnant. Finally on Friday, I was taken down to have a scan and afterwards was told that there was no hope. The medical staff wanted me to stay in hospital, but your dad was so distraught that he discharged me early and took me back to my mum's.

In the parking lot, when we got to the car, he had trouble opening the passenger door so he started kicking it in. He kicked so hard that it caved in and then was permanently shut. It was a three-door car, so from then on, everyone had to access the car through the driver's door. To me it was a permanent reminder of the tragedy of your death and a symbol of how deeply your dad grieved.

So your arrival in my womb was planned and greeted with joy and hope, but your departure brought grief and despair and really rocked the faith of Leroy and me. The baptism was cancelled as I was too ill in hospital to attend and your dad was too distressed to go through with it at that time. It was a very dark day. Of course, after you lose a baby your hormones are all over the show so I was very emotional, weepy, and very down. I was also very worried about your dad, who kind of retreated into himself; he just lay on the bed in a darkened room for a couple of days after I came out of hospital and did not really want to speak to anyone. I had to get up and carry on with life even though I was still bleeding heavily; after all, I had three other children who needed my attention. I think for the next few months, I kind of carried on regardless of what had happened. I was just kind of numb and I got through by focusing on what I had to do each day and on my other responsibilities. I prayed a lot and watched your dad anxiously as I was really worried that this might be the thing that made him take a drink to ease his pain and confusion. He stayed sober and kept his faith in God, which is a miracle.

To this day, I cannot truly understand why I miscarried. Of course, there may well be physiological reasons. I was told by the hospital that they don't investigate those unless a woman has more than three miscarriages and I "only" had two. It was more that I could not understand why God had allowed it. In the end, I just accepted it and came to see that it gave me a greater discernment into the nature of God and some of the false teachings that are around in the Christian church today. We don't speak and make God act—He is God. Period! The question I now ask when bad stuff happens is "Why Not Me?" I realize that God has not given or promised me a charmed, successful, healthy, wealthy life. He has given me eternal life. In heaven, my life will be grief and suffering free, but here on earth, not so. So I have a hope for the future, but here I have the same struggles and trials that everyone has. The difference is that God gives me strength and grace for each day.

Anyway, enough of all that. You were wanted here, but God chose to take you to be with him and although I suffered much anguish at the time, I accept it now.

Goodbye.

Love,
Your Mother
xxxx

P.S. Your dad did eventually get baptized in a swimming pool near where we lived. Your sister Sally got baptized at the same time along with your dad's mum. Our faith was shaken, but is now stronger than ever and God has indeed been good to us.

LETTER 14

How Blind Can Parents Be?

Dear Sally,

After I had my second miscarriage, I carried on with life in a bit of a daze. I was granted early retirement from teaching on the grounds of ill health. This in itself was a miracle as it is extremely difficult to get early retirement due to a stress-related illness. I had been teaching for twenty-two years and it was my life. Now what?

Life continued, of course, and there were a few highlights and some very lowlights.

Do you remember the plaited hair extensions? You asked me to pay for you to have them done. I couldn't, so you asked your dad and on this occasion (it was Christmastime), he sent you eighty pounds and you spent the lot on having a friend's mum put in the extensions. I think that they hurt you when you slept to begin with, but you persevered. You got into trouble at school, but I backed you. You won the argument and were allowed to keep them. Initially they suspended you and wanted to make you remove them before returning, but we argued that as you tied them back for school, you were complying with the rules, which did not state that braided hair extensions were not allowed.

I also had laser surgery on my eyes to correct my extreme shortsightedness. It was painful and did not work properly the first time so I had to have it redone, but overall, I think that it has been worth it. As I write this now, I am not wearing glasses although ten years on, I do need them for driving and shopping (can't read the labels!).

Daniel came home and left again—a few times.

There is one thing that happened during this time that really upset me and now that I know more about what happened on that night, I am mortified. You were out and rang and asked me if you could go and sleep over at a friend's house. The friend was a new one and I was not sure about you staying with her family; the phone-call was dodgy and I told you to come home. You did not come home, so I started to worry. I rang the friend's home and it appeared that they thought that the two of you were at our house. In the end, both of our families were out searching for you and we contacted the police. At 3 a.m. the police found you and brought you home. You had ended up near the house where Daniel was, by then, living. You were totally wasted, drunk as a skunk, and hardly coherent.

My first reaction was total relief that you had been found and that you were safe. My second reaction was fear. Because I had thrown out Daniel for drinking and taking drugs, I feared that if you continued in this way, I would have to apply the same rule to you and then I would have lost both of you. I wanted to make sure that you never pulled a stunt like that again so I grounded you for three months. For the first week, you were grounded to your room and after that you were grounded to the house. This meant that you had to come home from school and you were not allowed out at night. At first, you were not allowed out at the weekend, but after a few weeks, I allowed you to be out until a 4p.m. curfew.

I am so sorry that I did not persevere in trying to find out what really happened on that night and that I was not really there for you and that you did not feel that you could tell me what actually transpired. You have since told me and I am horrified. At the time, you did tell me that you got into a car with two older guys, but you did not elaborate; you made it sound like some kind of drinking joy ride. My sweet little girl lost her virginity that night and she did not consent. What kind of mother doesn't instinctively know that something like this has happened? Well, obviously the kind of mother that I am! Just know that if I had known I would have pursued and prosecuted the offenders. They would now be on the sex offender's register. You were only fourteen. It must have been so tough dealing with that on your own and there is no doubt that it will have an effect on the rest of your life. Sally, that is so like you. You keep things to yourself and even now you push me away when I try to be there for you. Now, I have to accept that you are a grown-up and let you go, but then you were a child and I should have been there for you.

Now that your little sister, Lilly, is a teenager, I am really trying to keep the lines of communication open with her, but it is hard because you guys reach an age of not wanting to talk to your mothers. I truly did not intend it to be like this. When I had children, I dreamed of being the parent that could talk about anything. Nothing would be taboo. I wanted to be the kind of parent that my children could be honest with and could confide in. I wanted to be a safe person to confide in. I don't think that you view me as that kind of person. I am safe to shout at, but not to confide in. All I can do now is assure you of my love and care for you both at that time and forever.

At the end of your grounding, we booked a flight to go to Canada as a family. This was a real highlight. I remembered all the good times we had there when you and Daniel were little and it was somewhere Leroy had always wanted to travel. We also bought a ticket for Daniel, even though he had come back to live with us and then left home again. Yet, again, it was a good holiday and brings back good memories for me as I hope it does for you. There were still some tough times with Daniel, but it is a good memory for me and I hope that you see it as a time when we tried to strengthen the bonds of our blended family. Leo was not with us, which was a shame, but maybe makes up for the Florida trip that you two missed out on. He was given the option of coming, but as we now know was too far into drugs, to commit to come along with us. Daniel ended up staying with my sister and her family for a couple of months and I was really hopeful that this was a new beginning for him.

I hope that you can see through this that my desire was for us to be together as a family and that this was also the desire of Leroy despite the glitches We have had many failings as parents, but have not failed in our desire for you to be fulfilled and happy and secure. More than anything nowadays, our desire is to see you fully commit your life to God and trust in him. We are mere humans and fail often, but he never fails us.

All my love,

Mum

xxxx

LETTER 15

The Yoyo Years Continue

Dear Daniel,

You returned from Canada and although I had a few misgivings because you immediately took up with your old friends, everything seemed to be going well. You even managed to go into school and take a couple of exams, following which, you got a job in a local factory. I started to notice odd things about your behavior and confronted you a few times, but you always denied taking drugs or drinking. At times I thought I was going mad.

Although the evidence before my eyes was compelling me to believe that you were back drinking and taking drugs, I had no hard proof and I truly did not want it to be true. One day, Sally found a dope pipe on a chair in the living room, which she gave to Leroy and me. We were then confronted with evidence and had to make a decision. You did not deny it this time and in fact, one day, I dropped you off at a mate's house and you actually screamed at me and said that you had been taking drugs all along even in Canada and that it wasn't so bad. You had fooled everyone including me. Taking drugs was not wrong; the fault was mine. I was a bad mother. All the other mothers did not mind their sons using cannabis, only me. That was the instant that my heart hardened toward you as I saw the utter hatred and revulsion in your eyes toward me.

We did not kick you out on the spot, but gave you a few weeks to find somewhere else to live. You seemed confident that you could find somewhere. It was a very, very sad time for me. I felt like I had finally lost you and that you absolutely hated me and hated everything I stood for. I felt completely deceived. We went away for a week's holiday to my mum's in Wales and when we returned, you came round and asked to come back and live. You said you had no money and that you had been sleeping rough.

At first, I would not allow you into the house. I made you some food, but would not let you come in. Finally, I let you into the kitchen and tried to persuade you to seek help for your drug and alcohol misuse. You said that if I let you come back home, you would get help. I said if you get help, I will let you come back home. Quite honestly, I did not believe you and I was sick of your promises. It was a catch-22. I offered to ring up and get you a bed for the night at a hostel and said that we could then talk in the morning. You refused and kept insisting that you wanted to come back home. I was too scared to let you stay even though I wanted with all my heart to say yes. It was one of the hardest things I have ever done, but I did not let you stay that night. You went outside and smashed up some outdoor furniture and after what seemed like an eternity, left. I was shaking with fear and total grief. I felt a complete and utter failure as a mother, in fact, as a human being. I did not sleep all night and I wanted to die. I kept thinking of you outside, alone, nowhere to go and I felt physically, mentally, and emotionally sick. My whole body was in a state of shock. I was racked with anguish. I did not know how I could go on. So if you thought that I sighed a sigh of relief when you finally left, popped off to my nice comfy bed with a hot chocolate, and fell promptly into a deep and satisfied sleep, awaking the next morning with a smile on my face, you are gravely mistaken.

You survived the night and I survived the night and you went back to live at your mate's house. In all of this, I don't know if you remember, but I actually paid your board at your mate's house; you did not live there for free. In fact, when we had gone to Wales after asking you to leave, I had given you money to give to your friend's mum and you had told me that you were going to stay with her whilst we were away. It turned out that you had in fact taken the money and spent it and had planned on coming back and living in the house whilst we were away. I discovered that the garage door had been left unlocked on the inside, but I locked it before we left. This was another of those occasions when you screamed abuse at me and told me that I was a useless mother. You told me that all your cousins smoked weed and that their mothers let them. This was news to me and I was gutted to think that you had been smoking weed whilst at my sister's house in Canada with one of her boys. I felt totally deceived. Of course, when I talked to my sister, she had not known about it, so she had been deceived, too. However, you were right; she did not kick out her son for taking drugs. You also kept telling me that Leo used drugs, but he was allowed to stay with us when he came for visits. Again I tried to catch him at it, but never succeeded. He always denied it and we never found any drugs on him. He was also compliant when he came to stay and didn't swear at me or refuse to help out. Of course, you were right, and he was in fact getting deeper and deeper into drugs. It must have seemed a total travesty of justice that he was allowed to stay with us on visits, but you were not allowed to sleep at the house. Honestly, if we had ever caught him, he would not have been allowed to visit.

Shortly after this I found out that I was pregnant again. This time I did not lose the baby and your little brother was born the following May. In a way, I felt that God was giving me another son, so that this time I could do things right. This son would stay home, and as it has turned out, I expect he will live with us into our old age, if we live to see it. Time went on and you managed to get a job at a garage, tire-fitting trucks and I hoped that the discipline of working would get you on track. Of course, through all of this, I was praying for you night and day.

Daniel, over the next couple of years we had our ups and downs—mostly downs. You lost your job and went on the dole. I helped you to fill in all the paperwork to get a council flat and again, I hoped that this would give you what you wanted: a place of your own where you could live as you pleased. Leroy and I paid for the whole place to be carpeted and bought paint so that you could redecorate it. We made sure that you had all the essentials of kitchen equipment and basic furniture. I always felt that whatever we did for you was never enough, and this was no exception. After you lost your job, you seemed to give up on trying and hated the fact that I would never give you hard cash. If you said you had no money for electricity, I would go down and put money on your electricity card. If you said you had no food, I would take you down to the supermarket and pay for food of your choice. This used to make you very angry, as all you really wanted was the cash.

It seemed that all the hopes I had were gone and life was becoming increasingly hard for me. At times, we seemed to start to have a relationship again, but mostly it was just deteriorating. You refused to come for Christmas and would not walk down the street with me or call me mum. It culminated with you starting to steal from me again and following that, I decided not to let you into the house. A showdown with Leroy ensued and it ended with you head-butting him. He lost a tooth and we had a restraining order put on you. What a mess.

One day, I went into Hanley town center with Nana and we were in a McDonalds; you came in with a friend. A surge of emotion went through me. I was so happy to see you and see that you looked well, but so sad that I could not speak to you. All I wanted to do was jump up and hug you, but I was too scared. I had not seen you for months.

Everything seemed hopeless, but I continued to love you with all my heart, even though it was breaking. I prayed for you night and day.

Love,

Mum

xxxx

LETTER 16

More Teenage Girl Stuff

Dear Sally,

After our first holiday to Canada with Leroy, we returned to England and life seemed to go on as normal for you: you went to school, you came to church with us and you went out with your friends both from school and from church. I suspected a few times that you had been drinking, but of course, you always hotly denied it. Daniel came back to live with us when he returned from Canada and it all looked as though things were going to work out, but it was not to be. After a while he started using dope again and naturally he got careless one day and left his pipe on a chair in the living room. You found it and gave it to me. Maybe if I had found it, I would have just thrown it away and said nothing, but as you found it, I was faced with having to have another confrontation. You kept asking me what I was going to do about it. It was obvious that Daniel was lying to us again. Leroy and I discussed the situation and decided to confront Daniel and ask him to find somewhere else to live. It was truly one of the saddest days of my life, as I so wanted to believe that he had given up.

Anyway, that is really part of my journey as his mother not really about you except in this instance, you were behind his exposure. I am sure that in time, he would have been careless again and it would have been the end of the road for him living with us anyway. So it was back to you, Lilly, Leroy, and I living together. I was absolutely devastated at the turn of events and I am not sure how I kept on going, but I did.

Then I found out that I was pregnant again.

Lilly had started to go to preschool for a couple of hours in the afternoon and one day I was so tired and felt so sick that I went to bed when she was there. I woke up and heard the phone ringing. It was the preschool wanting to know where I was. This was unheard of—I never went to bed in the afternoon, and although my nickname could truly be *little miss late,* it was never because I was asleep in bed at home. It was usually because I was rushing about somewhere trying to fit too much into my day.

I had already been to the doctor because my periods had stopped and he had assured me that I was not pregnant because I was going through an early menopause. Still, I felt so awful that on the way home from picking up Lilly, I bought a home pregnancy kit and found to my amazement/dismay/excitement/joy/despair that I was indeed pregnant again at forty-four years old. Leroy was over the moon and you were also quite excited at the prospect of another sibling. I, of course, was extremely worried that I would have another miscarriage, but this time, I went full term and Callum was the result.

Things were not, however, all hunky dory at our household. Leroy and I had become Christians, but we were still imperfect human beings and imperfect parents. We still had our ups and downs and you more than anyone would have been party to these at this time. From soon after Callum's birth, Leroy started to work away from home again and was away all week. I seem to remember that at this time, we spent quite a lot of time together. I often used to pick you up from school after I had picked up Lilly from school and the four of us—you, Lilly, Callum, and I—would go around together. Strangers often assumed that Callum was your son and my grandson. Daniel was living nearby, but you two kept your distance, apart from getting together once or twice when your dad came up to visit.

We moved house again and one night Leroy and you had some sort of disagreement about computer memory. The upshot of this was that Leroy left for work the next morning and gave me an ultimatum. He said that you would have to leave or he would leave me. I remember the sick feeling in my stomach returning with a vengeance; just when I thought things were on an even keel something like this would happen. On this occasion, I remember telling you that if push came to shove, I would stick with you. Do you remember that? I really could not understand why Leroy seemed to react like this when people disagreed with him. His solutions were always so drastic: black and white, with no inbetween. Of course, now I realize that he is on the autism spectrum so this explains much of how he reacts when there is a disagreement. You were very argumentative and you were a teenager so of course, were always positive that you were right and you were both dogged in your opinions. The relationship has always been a very hard one for both of you and although Leroy had apologized for his outburst when you were twelve, the matter did not seem to have been resolved for you. It was as though you still had a point to prove. (Of course, you realize that neither he nor I had any real idea of what you had been through and were coping with on your own. Maybe if we had, things would have been different.)

Fortunately I was not forced to make the choice of asking you to leave or standing up to Leroy as he had a week to think things through. He backed down from his ultimatum and you resolved your differences. It was a very tense week for me because I did not want to lose either of you and I love you both dearly. One of the things that I would still love to see happen between the two of you is total reconciliation and respect for each other.

I am finding now that a man and a teenage daughter is a potent combination, Leroy is your stepdad so it was even more complicated, but I notice that the same undercurrents are present between him and Lilly who is his own flesh and blood. Men seem to kind of expect that their daughters are perfect, obedient, and share with them the exact same opinions and beliefs. Any divergence in opinion is seen as insolence. I guess it is not just a dad thing; it is a parent thing. After all, we have been in the world a lot longer that you guys and we have weighed up life and come to our own considered conclusions about what is important and what is not. When we find out that our offspring have a different view, it is very hard to swallow. I feel it equally with my sons and daughters, but I think men are much more inclined to allow their sons to *live their own lives* and *be men,* but are much more protective over their daughters, have much higher expectations of them, and don't allow them to *live their own lives* and *be women.*

Believe it or not, there was some good stuff during this time. We had holidays, Centre Parks (one of your friends came, too) Cornwall and Canada again. You took your GCSEs (General Certificate of Education) and got fantastic grades. You had your Year Eleven Leaving do and looked absolutely fabulous in black and red. Do you remember those shoes? Red with six-inch heels!

So, things were starting to settle down for us as a family. Although Daniel was not living with us, he had a job and somewhere to stay. As his eighteenth birthday had approached, I helped him to apply for a council flat, which he was granted. Unfortunately, things at this time went badly wrong for him. He lost his job and did not cope with having a flat. Leroy and I helped him financially by buying him things to help him do up the flat, but it seems his life was spiraling out of control. One day he came round and I would not let him in because he had stolen money from me on the previous visit. I gave him food, but there was an argument at the door. I had to get Leroy involved and Daniel ended up head butting Leroy and Leroy lost one of his front teeth. We went to the police and a court order ensued. As usual, my solution to a family problem was to divide and rule. In 2004, I feared that because Daniel was on an order from the court not to come near Leroy or I or the house, he would get at us by getting at you. He had started to phone you and ask you to meet him near the house. I knew he would be asking you for money or help in some way and did not see how you were going to be able to cope. I could not move and I could not see how I could stop him. I did not want to set you against your own brother and knew your loyalties would be very much divided. Leroy was working away. I was very consumed with the practicalities of looking after a toddler and a very tricky five-year-old on my own, so I asked my sister if you could go and stay with them for a while.

So after completing your GCSEs, you ended up going to Canada. This was something that I thought you really wanted to do as when we were there earlier in the year, you had talked about wanting to return to go to Bible School there. This was not the same as when you went to Nana's. It was to protect you and you seemed excited and happy about going. It was more of an adventure.

I feel I must put a word in here about your Auntie Lina and Uncle Peter. Since I was fifteen, she has been a *long distance* sister to me. We have not even lived on the same continent since I was sixteen. Despite the distance, we have kept in touch and made opportunities to get together as family. When I was a single parent and we made those trips to Canada, it was a wonderful oasis in a troubled time. When we went with Daniel in 2002 and they offered to give him a fresh start that was a labor of love. Finally, when this situation arose, they offered to open their home for you to stay with them. When I made a will shortly after my separation from your father, I named them as your guardians in the event of my death. They have always looked out for you and Daniel and made a special effort to get to know all of my children. When they were living in Canada, my sister was always only a phone-call away from me.

So it was that you ended up going there again and, like my mum, your aunt's stipulation was that you had to have something to do. Leroy paid for you to do courses at the college where your Uncle Peter was teaching and we were careful to stick to the terms of your visa. He also paid for you to stay at Aunty Lina's and I kept a record of the bank statements, which showed the payments going out to them each month. I was so glad I did this because later on, when we were applying for permanent residency in Australia, I needed these bank statements to prove that you were dependent on us during this time.

You stayed with your auntie and uncle for eight months and during that time got a real desire to actually go and live there. When you came back to us you were in the process of applying for a student visa to go and study over there. You had two colleges in mind. I was quite sad, but understood your desire as Leroy and I had actually started to apply to go and live in Canada so we understood its appeal.

Back at the ranch, I had been finding life unbearable. Leroy was working in London. I was home now with Lilly who was in year 1 at school and hating every minute of it and Callum who was a toddler and very attached to me. It was a very lonely time for me. I was now totally estranged from Daniel and you were in Canada. I felt like a single parent again. This may explain my next major decision.

Love,

Mum

xxxx

LETTER 17

999 and What Followed

Dear Sally,

Wow, your life certainly has had its moments! This was no exception. There you were, back from Canada, going to work in Crewe, biding your time as you were making application to go back and study full time in Canada. Things had become unbearable for me living near Daniel and we had decided to move to Wales. You were not excited about that, but relieved that you were not going to live there for long as you were set on going back to Canada.

During the time that you were in Canada, we had made moves to be reconciled once again to Daniel. Leroy wrote him a letter saying that he had forgiven him for the assault and at the same time, I bought a bag of groceries and went round to his flat. We had come to some sort of truce, but I still felt very uneasy and often felt threatened when Daniel asked me for money and I refused. It was breaking my heart to see him in such a state. I tried to help him as much as I could with groceries and electricity tokens, but what he actually wanted was money that I would not give him. I dreaded every unexpected knock at the door.

It was in this situation that we put our house on the market. We found a house in Wales that we wanted to buy and I enrolled Lilly to start school in Prestatyn the following school year. For some reason, the house that we were going to buy fell through and so I was busy trying to find somewhere to rent in Wales. Then it happened. One day whilst looking at rental properties in Wales, I had a phone-call from you. You were in pain and had come home from work. (When you came back from Canada, you immediately set about getting yourself a job. This is a quality I have always admired. You do not sit around waiting for work to come your way.) The tone of your voice worried me, so I quickly got in the car and came back home with Lilly and Callum.

When I arrived you were still in pain, but we didn't know what it was. You took some painkillers and lay curled up in bed. I really did not know what to do and did not know how serious the pain was. At this point, you did not want me to take you to hospital so I went to bed and in the early hours of the morning, you called out to me. By this time, you were in agony and I decided to ring for an ambulance as I realized that you needed emergency medical care. When the ambulance arrived, I became quite angry because the medical team did not seem to be taking your pain seriously and insinuated that maybe you just had a hangover and upset stomach from partying. I assured them that you had not been out the night before and that you did indeed need to go to hospital. I was already distressed because I could not go with you, as there was nobody that I could call to come over in the middle of the night to look after Callum and Lilly. It was a very tense few hours for me wondering if you were okay. The hospital rang me and said that you had acute appendicitis and that you were undergoing emergency surgery. At this point, I rang Leroy and asked him to return from London, as I could not see how I was going to be able to get to the hospital and visit you, as children were not allowed on the ward.

So, my precious daughter, your life was saved by the surgery and your emergency also meant that Leroy was spared death, injury, or at the very least trauma, because instead of getting on the tube to work, he went to Euston station in the very early hours of the morning to get the train back to Stoke-on-Trent. The tube he would have taken was the one that was blown up on the morning of July 7, 2005 in London. God works in mysterious ways.

The next few weeks were very traumatic for you especially, but also for me. I originally thought that you would be out of hospital in a few days and then would recover at home and be fine after about two weeks. This is what the hospital told me. Shortly after your operation, Leroy was back in London and he rang me one day to say that he had been offered a job in Australia; he wanted to accept, but had told the company that he would need to discuss it with me. Something just came over me and I said no need to discuss the job with me, take it and we will go to Australia for a year. At the time I couldn't believe what I was saying, but somehow in my heart, I felt it was right.

Leroy came back at the weekend and visited you in hospital. He told you about the job and asked you if you wanted to come with us. Although you had been applying to go back to Canada, it seemed there were some complications, as the colleges wanted you to have "*A*" Levels for you to be entered for their degree courses. Whatever the case, you said yes to Leroy and seemed quite excited at the prospect of going to Australia instead. You told us that it was somewhere you had always wanted to go and at the time, I think it gave you something to look forward to.

However after your operation there were complications. I really felt for you at this time as your body really suffered. You did not come out of the anesthetic well and subsequently, your wounds became infected and your lung collapsed. This meant that you were in and out of hospital for six weeks. On one occasion, two days after you had been re-admitted to hospital, I had to stand at the nurses' station and shout for attention until finally a consultant came to see you at your bed. It was fortunate that I was an obstinate, pestering mother at this point because he had to perform emergency surgery at your bedside! Later, when your lung collapsed, you were put in what seemed like a geriatric ward for twenty-four hours, which was really shocking for me. At this point, I became really concerned about you and about the care you were receiving at the hospital, as it was really hard for me to stay strong and not to show my distress.

It was also very hard because we were selling our house and I was packing up everything single-handedly as Leroy continued to work in London. I was also visiting you every day in hospital and having to find people to look after Lilly and Callum, as they were not allowed on the ward. Because we were no longer moving to Wales, I was faced with a mountain of stuff to dispose of. Looking back, if I had thought about it a bit more, I would have put some of our furniture in a container and had it shipped to Australia, but I just moved continents the way I remembered my parents had always moved continents. I gave away everything we had, apart from one car and a beautiful leather suite. I sold the car to a car dealer for a knockdown price and the leather suite I sold for a nominal figure to a couple I knew that needed furniture. The rest of the furniture I offered to Daniel and he chose another leather suite that we had, plus some lamps, a computer and a computer desk. In the end, he had a vanload of furniture and I felt good that we had been able to help him in that way. It had been some time since he had allowed me to go into his flat, but I hoped that this would make him more comfortable. The rest of the furniture I gave to a charity and some we gave to a church in a local town that we had been attending. I gave away all my personal possessions apart from a few photos, clothes, and sentimental trinkets that Daniel or you had given or made for me when you were little. A friend, Christy from the local church, offered to look after my piano and some African artifacts.

Those few weeks were like a whirlwind for me. On the one hand, I was visiting you in hospital and sitting quietly with you beside your bed. I was extremely worried about your health and well-being and at one point, I even worried about your life itself. I am not sure if you realized at the time just how sick you were. The only positive side I could see was that it gave us an opportunity to spend time together. On the other hand, I was in the process of completely dismantling the house and all its contents whilst looking after a clingy toddler and an often distraught, six-year-old. Every time I got into my little car, I put in a few boxes of stuff, which I then took to local charity shops. Most of the stuff was very good quality and ranged from badminton racquets to telescopes, from dollhouses to electric drills and so it went on. I piled up goods of all description in the front porch and every time anyone came to the house, from Avon lady to postman, I asked them to take something with them.

It was also an exciting time as I sat in hospital with you, and we talked about the adventure of going to Australia. I finally felt at peace about moving away from Daniel. This way I could actually tell him where I was going. I could give him my address and he would be able to contact me if he wanted to. I am very grateful to one particular friend, Christy, who put herself out to look after Lilly and Callum and also agreed to be my contact person with Daniel. She made it possible for me to visit you every day.

Of course, this leads me on to the real reason for this letter. Leroy's contract in Australia commenced on September 12. He was advised that he should be there for at least a few days before that date to give him a chance to get over his jetlag and acclimatize to Australia. He was given 457 visas for his family and you were included in those visas as his dependent. As you were under eighteen, I had to get written permission from your dad for you to go and live in Australia. This I did, but then the doctors advised us that you would not be fit to fly in September due to your collapsed lung. I was faced with another impossible decision. You wanted me to stay with you in England until December and Leroy was insistent that I fly with him, Lilly, and Callum in September. It just so happened that his parents, his brother, and sister-in-law were due to go on holiday to Australia in December and they were more than happy for you to travel with them. Nana was excited to have you stay with her whilst you recovered and also my cousin Carol said that she would love you to come and stay with her. It seemed like the perfect solution to me. I knew you would be in safe hands with Nana and your Aunty Carol, and I knew that you would not have to fly alone.

You really wanted me to stay with you, but I could not. We did not have anywhere to live as we had sold the house. We spent the last couple of weeks in the United Kingdom living at Nana's and as you know, she has a small two-bedroom bungalow. Leroy could not have taken Lilly and Callum to Australia, as he would have to go to work every day so they would have had to stay in the UK as well. I know now that you felt abandoned again, but I truly felt like I was making the best decision for everyone. Less than three months after we flew to Australia, you followed us, arriving on December 1· 2005. Looking back, I think it was definitely better that way, as those first three months here in Australia were awful. I don't think we would have survived as a family unit if you had been part of that extreme stress. Nevertheless, this does not minimize the fact that you felt abandoned and that you felt like I had chosen Leroy over you. What can I say except that I chose what I considered to be the only practical path that was open to me, one that catered adequately to everyone's needs. Believe me, I was very sad to have to leave you behind; it tore my heartstrings, but I truly felt that it was best for everyone. You had the chance to recuperate in peace and quiet and I had the chance to get over here and help Leroy, Lilly, and Callum to settle into the new country.

I hope that you will forgive me for leaving you with the feeling of abandonment and that you will realize that you were not abandoned, just left in safe hands for a time. I have never abandoned you in my heart.

Love,

Mum

xxxx

LETTER 18

Different Continents

Dear Daniel,

It is now six-and-a-half years since I came to Australia. It has been a bumpy ride to say the least. There has been excitement, exhaustion, bewilderment, bemusement, panic, peace, relief, regret, fear, faith, despair, delight, sorrow, and joy. I have gone through a rollercoaster of emotions.

When we first arrived here, I was very, very excited—totally exhausted, but nevertheless excited. It really was a new beginning for me. Everything was new; even the grass here looked different. I had never seen anything like it; it looked plastic and artificial and even felt quite rubbery and bouncy when you walked on it. The other spin-off was that I was no longer afraid to open the door when I heard a knock. I could walk down the street without feeling that people were looking at me and judging me for being the woman that could not control her children and kicked out her son before he was fifteen. No one here knew me or of our family history and I could start again. I could start again without feeling like I was running away because I had a legitimate reason to be here. I had been able to let you know where I was going, whereas originally, I had been planning on moving away and not divulging my whereabouts.

You did not know, but my desperation had become so great that I had been planning on selling the house in England and moving to Wales without leaving you my new address. I did not plan to lose contact. I was going to regularly write to you, buy you food, and hopefully visit you, but I was not going to live dreading the knock on my door and seeing you on the other side totally wasted, angry, and maybe battered. That was how bad the situation had become for me. I had been dreading this move, but could not see any other solution. I needed to be able to live in peace. Whether moving away in those circumstances would have brought me peace, I do not know, but God thought differently and he provided another more honorable way for me to leave.

Leroy was offered the job in Australia, initially for twelve months, with a promise of at least two years work. He would be able to live at home with us and be a proper father and husband. Sally had decided not to go back to Canada to continue her studies, but to come with us and she was just young enough to be included on Leroy's visa, it being a couple of months before her eighteenth birthday. In an ideal and different world and set of circumstances, we would have also been bringing you and Leo, but as we all know, we do not live in an ideal world. My hope and constant prayer was that with me in Australia, and your own dad still drinking, you would finally have to face the reality of your own situation and come to your senses. In AA, they call it reaching rock bottom. There is, of course, a risk in this as no one really knows where their own or someone else's rock bottom is, and there are some who reach the ultimate rock bottom of death before they call out for and receive help. I always hoped and believed that this would not be the case for you. I had faith that one day, you would accept Jesus as your Savior and become an ambassador for him. I also believed and hoped that one day you and your stepbrother would be able to come to Australia, but I realized that this would only happen in miraculous circumstances.

Before we left England, I had been struggling to get through each day. I spent most of my time at home with Callum and Lilly. The restraining order against you was lifted and we had some kind of reconciliation, but all was not well. You were still choosing to live a lifestyle that I found extremely frightening and confusing. I could hardly bear to see the choices that you were making. I longed for you to turn around and reject the lifestyle of alcohol, drugs, and fighting that you had chosen. Every time there was a knock at the door during the week, my heart sank in case it was you, back for another argument, back to have another pop at me, back to tell Lilly and Callum that I was a bad mother and that they should not listen to me. Yet, at the same time, I was glad to see you because that meant that you were still alive.

Of course, you were also there to ask for money, food, and a shower. You always were concerned with your cleanliness! You also used to bring me your washing; usually by the time you brought it, my guess is that you had nothing clean left to wear, as it usually took me all day to wash and dry it. This I liked to do; it made me feel like a real mother, and it made me feel like I could actually do something for you. I also loved to go to the supermarket and buy you food. Often I bought you cigarettes and electricity tokens for your meter. Doing these things also made me feel like a real mother. These were normal things to do in a mother-son relationship that was far from normal. Money was always the sticking point. I rarely gave you money as I suspected that you would spend it on alcohol or drugs. All the advice I received from Al

Anon and other agencies was telling me not to even provide you with
food, as that would then free up any money you had for alcohol and
drugs, but as a mother, I just could not deny you food. At times, I had to
deny you access to the house and during the time of the restraining
order, I had no contact with you at all. That was indeed a dreadful time.
I died inside. The only thing that kept me alive at that time was God.
My faith in him was unshakable. He was my rock and my foundation. I
held on to the belief that one day God would bring you to your senses
and that he would lift you up out of the miry pit that you were in.
Meanwhile, I could not bear to see you in that pit. When we met, the
hate and anger you had toward me was almost tangible; it exuded from
every pore in your body. There seemed to be no answer to our relationship dilemma. You wanted to live at home. I wanted you to live at
home, but I could not allow you to live at home whilst you continued in
your lifestyle as I now had two young children at home. You kept
promising me that you would change (give up taking drugs and drinking alcohol) if you lived at home, but I would not let you live at home
until you had given up taking drugs and drinking alcohol and I saw
some evidence of this. Most of our arguments revolved around this
issue.

I did not trust you to stay away from drugs and alcohol because of all
the times in the past when I had let you come to live back at home and
you had continued to take drugs and consume alcohol and I had to ask
you to leave again. Each time this happened, a piece of my heart was
broken off. Although you promised to give up alcohol and drugs, you
took every opportunity to tell me that I was unreasonable and that I was
not a real mother because proper mothers put up with their sons whatever their behavior and accepted them no matter what. All your friends,
you said, were just as bad as you and they had not been kicked out. It
was only I, the abnormal, crazy one, who thought cannabis was so bad.
I was not worthy to be called a mother and at one point, you refused to
call me mum. You often screamed obscenities at me and seemed to take
delight in mocking everything about me. Many times you said that you
would like to take me on "Oprah" to put your case, and then the whole
world would see what a useless mother I was. I would be judged and
you would be vindicated. You never did, of course, but the total scorn
in your attitude hurt me beyond measure. All I ever wanted to do was to
take you in my arms and love you better, rock you to sleep, and everything would be all right in the morning, but life is not like that. Issues
have to be addressed and lives have to be changed.

Yet, there were moments when we connected. Just inside the doorway, I had a little imitation telephone table with a seat. On one side was a little drawer with a cupboard underneath. In the cupboard, I kept "Chick" tracts. They were little comic strip tracts that gave the gospel in a short, eye-catching form. You often used to sit there on your way in or out of the house and flick through them, sometimes asking me questions about the content, but mostly just reading them. I hoped and prayed that their message would get through to you that there was hope and a different way of living.

Sometimes, you came to the door and there was a real glimmer of fear in your eyes and you would tell me about the weird things that you saw at night and ask me how you could make them go away. I would tell you to pray and call on God's name and ask him to reveal himself to you. You told me that you had waking visions of an angelic being. This being would appear in your room and just when you started to feel safe, the face of the angelic being would change into a demonic, sinister face and the creature would laugh at you. I do not know if these were drug-induced hallucinations of yours or even if you remember those occasions now. They made me remember the little frightened boy who could not be upstairs at night if I was downstairs or downstairs if I was upstairs. You were the same boy who ended up sleeping in my bedroom in London because he was too scared to sleep in his own; the same boy who at twelve, when you moved into your own loft bedroom, after I married Leroy, still had to be reassured and settled into bed with music and soft lights. Even then, I often sang "Silent Night" to you at your request.

On rare moments, we would even catch each other's eye and laugh about a funny event or happening, and in that instant we would connect and I would feel that I was your mum again. The instant would disappear almost as soon as it had appeared and the hostile eyes would return, but that glimmer warmed my broken heart and I knew that there was a broken relationship worth saving and that there could one day be reconciliation.

Leroy was working away from home in London before we left England and I hardly saw him. He arrived home late on Friday night and was gone again on Sunday afternoon. Saturday he spent taking Lilly swimming, doing some grocery shopping, and preparing a sermon for Sunday morning. Sunday, we went to church, he preached, and I taught the small Sunday school class. Again, I had Callum with me. I usually had to carry him whilst I was teaching Lilly and the three or four other children who came to Sunday school. I actually felt like a single parent all over again, only this time I had one estranged teenager son—you— to deal with and also a teenage daughter, Sally, who had gone to Canada for a few months to be with my sister and thus escape the stress caused by our estrangement and was planning on returning there on a full-time basis. Australia might just be a chance to live a semi-normal family life again if even for just a year. So although I was desperately sad at the circumstances that would have forced me to leave the area where you were living and although I was devastated that my family life was not turning out the way I expected or hoped, I felt that God was giving me a chance to try to build a family the proper way in a new country.

On arrival, everything seemed new and different. Australia had never really been on my horizon; I was terribly ignorant of what to expect when I got here. Like most people in England, I knew about Bondi Beach, Sydney Opera House, Uluru (Ayers Rock), Alice Springs, Aborigines, boomerangs, walkabout, kangaroos, koalas, and convicts—but not much else.

I will never forget the first week we were here in Australia. The jet lag was like nothing I had ever experienced before or since. Not only were we utterly and totally exhausted and time confused from the trip, which actually took us three days as we left on Friday morning and arrived on Sunday evening, but it was also as if we had arrived on a different planet. This planet looked somewhat similar to the one we left and at least we could read the signs, but nothing was the same. It was frightening, as we had absolutely no idea where anything was. We were not met by anyone that we knew or could call. We wanted to sleep all day and were wide-awake all night, but even during the day, sleep evaded us as Callum seemed to be awake all the time and since he was only two-and-a-half, needed constant supervision. During that first week, we bought a map, hired a car, and found out where the nearest supermarket was. We also got Lilly into school. The company that had brought Lee over here gave him a week to get his bearings and he started work on the second Monday we were here. I also started the hunt for a new home for us as we only had three weeks booked in the house the company had arranged for us to rent. It was furnished, but we found out that most of the rental properties in Sydney are not. As a result, we also had to find furniture so that when we moved we would have something to sleep on, sit on, eat off, etc. We also had no plates or cutlery; in fact, we only had a few clothes, personal possessions, and toys for Callum.

Still, when I got here, I felt like part of me had been cut off—not an arm or a leg or anything that you could see, but part of me as a person—the part of me that is you. It had only been hanging by a thread before we left, but now I felt totally cut off. I could not be in control even if I wanted to. I could not rescue you, and I really had to leave you in the hands of God. I was happy that you knew where I was and I had not had to run away and hide. I was happy that some friends of mine (Christy and her husband) had told us that you could go there anytime if you wanted to e-mail me or get in touch for any reason. I was happy that they had also said that I could send any letters or gifts for you to their house and that they would deliver them to you. (After seeing the stairs behind the door to your upstairs flat on a couple of occasions, which were littered with weeks of unopened mail, I had visions of writing to you or sending you a gift and it lying there unopened for months on end.) I was happy that my cousin had promised me that she would be there for you, pray for you, ring you, and invite you over for meals and drive down and pick you up and take you to her home. She has acted like a godmother to you in the true sense of the word even though she is not your godmother.

I also felt that it was a new beginning for me, and that I could now do the job of parenting properly with the two youngest. I have always felt a failure in this area, like somehow I am swimming in the sea, but I don't know the strokes and can't see the shore. I guess this is partly because my own childhood was so institutionalized. I went from hostel to children's home to boarding school. I had very little experience of family life on which to draw. I now know that holiday parenting is not the same as the constant everyday parenting that I rarely experienced. In this, I can see that my ideas of family life were somewhat romanticized in my head. In the holidays, I would always want to please my parents, as I knew the time would be short and I would be back at the boarding school that I hated with a passion. Why ruin the holidays? I never told my parents how I felt about boarding school, I just accepted the way it was. Everyone else at boarding school hated being there, so I thought that boarding school was a way of life for families like mine. I really cannot remember ever having an argument with them of any kind. I cannot remember answering them back. I always remember accepting it when they said "no" to any request I might make, which would only be things such as "can we go swimming today?" I did not ask to do things that I already knew were not allowed.

The only thing I remember asking was why I could not attend the local mission school in Congo. This was a school run by the mission for local Congolese students and was part of their mission's work. My parents were not teachers there, but some of the other missionaries were. It seemed to me that if it was good enough for them, it was good enough for me. My parents' reasoning was that the lessons were taught in French and it was not run to British standards. They felt that I would be disadvantaged in my education if I was learning in a language other than my mother tongue.

Of course, having now been an educator myself, I know that this would in fact have highly advantaged me and would have forged intellectual pathways in my brain that would have improved my intellectual skills like almost nothing else, but like everything else, I accepted their reasoning and I believe they made their choices in good faith and wanting the best for me and my sister.

The point of me saying this is that I did not have any idea or any examples of how to resolve conflict in a family situation. It is still something I find very hard. Because I accepted my parents as the ultimate authority and generally wanted to please them, I could not understand when my own children did not accept my authority and did not want to please me. I did not know what to do. I was completely at a loss. So when you started experimenting with drugs and alcohol, I did not understand it when I told you that it was not acceptable that you continued. I did not understand it even on the simple levels when you were a younger child, I told you it was time to come in from playing, and you defied me. Now I realize that training is involved and that parenting requires training; obedience does not come naturally. While you were growing up, I was dealing with a lot of issues in my life. Living with alcoholism in the family is very difficult and damaging. After your father and I separated, I guess I felt very guilty that you and your sister only effectively had one parent and I think that this made me very soft with you in the earlier years as far as discipline and obedience were concerned. I did not teach you to respect me or indeed any authority.

What did I teach you? Only you can tell me that. I merely know I thought I was teaching you to think independently and to not take any guff from anyone. I thought I was teaching you that every human being was of equal value, regardless of his or her gender, race, age, or ability.

I thought I was teaching you that faith in God was an individual decision and that I could not decide for you either way. Because I had been at gunpoint myself, I was very strong on not allowing you to have any war toys (you never understood that one!). Sadly, I omitted to teach you respect and compliance with rules of home, school, and society. By that I mean I upheld them verbally, but did not enforce the home rules.

It is only now, after twenty-five plus years of parenting that I am beginning to realize what parenting is all about. I realize now that the early years are very important and that a child has to learn that no means no, but also that that is not the end of the world. Something that is not allowed now might be allowed when the child is older, or when the parents have enough money, or when the time is right. There are also occasions when a child might not be mature enough to understand a parent's decision and they just have to learn to accept that the decision is made in love and for a purpose. I also understand the importance of being a role model for your children. Children are going to find it difficult to resolve conflicts in their own lives if they have never seen conflicts resolved at home. I am now trying to show the younger children that when there is a conflict, when people disagree and even dispute and argue that afterwards, there can be reconciliation. Life can go on. It is not the end of the world. People are allowed to disagree and still get along. We don't always get our own way; we don't always get what we want. I find training children very hard. I just want it to be easy and for them to do what I expect without a fuss. I have had to learn that parenting requires hard work and almost single-minded dedication as well as love and good will. It involves hard decisions, especially when there is more than one child.

Safety is one of the overriding necessities. As parents, we have to keep our children safe, but then we also have to teach them how to keep themselves safe. This is one of the reasons that I felt Australia was going to enable me to be that role model to your younger brother and sister. I did not want them to see the conflict between us that was at that time unresolved. I did not want them to see the bitterness that you had for me or to see the total disregard for any discipline I tried to instill in them. You may not remember, but often you would tell them not to listen to me and that what I was teaching them was not true. One day around Christmastime, you paid us a visit. At the time, we had not told Lilly that Santa was not real. She was getting excited about Christmas and about what she would get from Santa. You laughed your head off and told her that Santa was not real and that she was not going to get anything from him. I was standing behind her, shaking my head and putting my finger up to my lips, silently asking you not to shatter her illusions. You took no notice and continued to say, "Santa is not real and neither is Jesus. Don't believe anything Mum tells you. You will find out that it is all lies."

This made me stop in my tracks although I was very angry. I realized that you had put a finger on my hypocrisy. Santa is indeed a fantasy figure, but Jesus is not. Here I was, I had become a Christian myself, and I was teaching my children to believe in a lie: Santa. I quickly redressed the situation and told Lilly that you were right about Santa and wrong about Jesus. Because of that day, Callum has never been brought up to believe in Santa. I hated being lied to above all else and here I was lying to my own children.

Every time you came into the house, I was scared that you would steal money. As soon as I saw you at the door, I would make a mental note of where my handbag was and I returned to my habit of keeping little or no change in my purse because of the occasions when you had stolen. I know that it was desperation and hunger that eventually turned you to stealing, but it started when you were young and wanted something that I did not have the money to buy or did not want you to have. I separated from your father because of fear and lies in an effort to provide you and Sally with a life without the overriding tension that comes with living with an alcoholic. I was now distancing myself physically from you in an effort to provide Sally, Lilly, and Callum with a life without fear and lies. I felt that with coming to Australia, at least I was able to do this honorably; there was another reason for leaving and it was nothing to do with you.

Leroy and I felt that God was leading us to Australia. I forsook everything else to do this. I forsook all my friends and the rest of my family, especially my mum and cousin, whom I have continued to miss on a daily basis. I missed you and always had a silent grief inside me as I thought about you and your situation, but I got on with my life and settling into a new country. I was accepted at face value and got a rare glimpse into what must make some people run away from home and become a missing person. I had the opportunity to start afresh, on a clean page, so to speak. Of course, I was not a missing person and have kept all my connections to my old life in England, but here I could be whoever I wanted to be and no one would know anything about my past unless I told them. It also symbolizes to me sometimes how it felt when I became a Christian. I became a new creation, and God forgave my past. Old things were behind me and everything was new.

So you see, every day and every night—literally twenty-four/seven—you were in my thoughts and prayers. I loved you from a distance. Did you feel it? I sent you letters and gifts and got news of you from my friends in Stoke. A couple of times, you e-mailed me; one in particular was suicidal. My heart was bleeding for you. Leroy and I both dreaded phone-calls to say that either you or Leo had died. Still life carried on and you survived.

But things were about to change, and the change could not have been better.

Love,

Mum

xxxx

LETTER 19

Our Australian Adventure Gets Serious

A) THE SCHOOL OF SIGNS AND WONDERS

Dear Sally,

I can't believe that I brought you to Australia just so that you could get involved in a cult and I truly believe that Sunrise Church has all the markings of a cult. I feel so guilty that I ever introduced you to the people from that awful place.

It is just like a wall has gone up between us. I cannot get through to you on any level whatsoever. There is nothing that I seem to be able to do that will get you to see sense. We are fighting to get permanent residency here in Australia and have been told that unless you leave the School of Signs and Wonders and go to a proper college, we have virtually no chance of being accepted for permanent residency here. This is not your mother talking, Sally, this is some random agent who helps people get visas in Australia. It has taken me months to prepare all the documentation to prove that you are our dependent. (Those bank statements from your time in Canada have come in handy, as they prove that we were supporting you whilst you were there.) We got over the first little glitch that because you did not fly with us on September 4, 2005, but instead flew on December 1, 2005, it meant that you were over eighteen when you arrived here. This initially caused a problem with you being included on Leroy's 457 visa, but we resolved that with medical evidence and proof that we paid for your ticket to come over here.

But then this—what was I to do? We had been told to take you off our application for permanent residency, but I would not. We came as a family and applied as a family. In this I put my foot down; I would not leave you off. There was too much at stake for me to leave you off the application, for it would mean that you would have had to apply on your own for residency. Based on your circumstances, you did not stand a chance of gaining it at that time, which meant that you would have had to leave the country in twenty-eight days. On the other hand, if we included you in the application and that resulted in us not getting permanent residency, it meant that we would all have had to leave the country in twenty-eight days.

Apart from all that, I was also very worried about what was happening to you. Sally. Sunrise church was playing with your mind, telling you not to listen to your parents, telling you not to believe anything that you had been taught about the Bible before attending their school, not to mention the obsession that they seemed to have with physical health and bodily training. I thought it was supposed to be a Bible School not a boot camp. They had no right to weigh you; no right to expect you to perform physical training tests; no right to make you attend prayer meetings at 6:00 a.m.; no right to tell you to "empty your mind"; no right to keep you so busy that you did not have time to think for your-self; no right to make you go on group "bonding" camps. I was not sure exactly what went on at these camps, but during one you were involved in a near fatal car accident, and during another you tore a tendon in your ankle and were forced to "claim your healing" and to continue with the three-day trek in the Blue Mountains. This was nothing short of negligence and abuse, but no matter what I said, you defended them and would not leave. They filled your head with such nonsense, saying you had the *gift* of interpreting dreams and sent you to work at the Mind, Body, and Soul Festival in a "Dream Interpretation" tent. Yes, I knew that God sometimes uses dreams and visions and that God gave insight to Joseph and Daniel to interpret the dreams of people in the Old Testament, but not in the same way that you were taught to inter-pret others dreams, with stock interpretations for certain dreams. This was not Christianity, but it fitted in with New Age Philosophy. I knew some people put a lot of stock in this philosophy, but at least they didn't pretend that it was Christianity.

I felt that I had lost you as a daughter. You were living with us, but were in constant opposition to us in the house. You belittled everything that we said and really wanted nothing to do with us. This made me feel so sad. If we got permanent residency and you decided to continue with the School of Signs and Wonders, I was going to have to ask you to live somewhere else, which I felt would be only fair to you and to us as the constant tension was not doing any of us any good. You would then be free to live the way you wanted to live, free from interference from us, and you would have every right to stay here as an individual in the country to which we brought you and which you love. I hoped that this way our relationship would improve and of course, one day, I hoped that you would see through the teachings of Sunrise Church.

I continued to love you.

Mum

xxxx

B) PERMANENT RESIDENCY AND ALL THAT JAZZ.

Dear Sally,

Well, what a miracle—now that really was a sign and wonder! We got permanent residency within three weeks of sending off our application—against all the odds. What an amazing feeling that was for me. I felt as though I was floating on air for days. I don't know how it felt for you, Sally, but I felt that somehow I had been vindicated for leaving you on the application and that God had honored my faithfulness in believing it was right to include you and not abandon you. If we had left you off, I believe that Sunrise Church would have somehow got you a visa as a religious worker and then you would have really been tied to them, almost like a slave, for two years. Anyway that was not the only reason I was elated, having lived for two years under the threat of having to leave the country with twenty-eight days notice had taken its toll and I was so relieved just to know that this was no longer hanging over us as a family. We could breathe easy. It also gave me a feeling that I was in the right place.

Getting permanent residency also freed you to stop being dependent on us for accommodation and for your very existence in Australia. You were and still are Sally Moran, Australian Permanent Resident, with the freedom to reside in Australia for the rest of your natural life, if you so wish. It also freed you to live life in your own place with your own rules.

As for getting older and wiser, even us *wrinklies* slip up from time to time. Getting permanent residency made Leroy and I a little rash (what a surprise!) and we went out and bought a house in the neighborhood far too quickly. As you know, it turned into a nightmare as we had really noisy neighbors, but fortunately for you that was not your problem. You had already started to look for somewhere to live with some friends and agreed to move out after we moved into our new house. I felt sad that you were moving out, but also relieved that there would be less tension in the house. It was good to see you settle into such a beautiful house nearby and everything seemed to be going well for you. I felt that because you were no longer in the house on a daily basis, we were able to get along in a more adult child and mother kind of way.

When it came time for your twenty-first birthday, I was so happy to be involved in your birthday party celebrations, even if you were anxious for us to leave early. I couldn't really understand why (well, I know that you think that I am the most embarrassing person in the world, but apart from that). I thought you would be glad that we were supporting you *on your own turf.* It was so funny. I remember you saying, "Mum, I am twenty-one and I am going to have a drink whether you like it or not."

I had fully expected you to have a drink and, in fact, I had seen crates of beer being brought into the house by your Sunrise Church friends. I remember saying, "Sally, you are twenty-one and this is your house not mine. You don't have to have my permission or approval."

I then realized that you were embarrassed to have a drink in front of Leroy and me, because of our stance on alcohol and, of course, the fact that Leroy was a drinking alcoholic for twenty-five years. In a way, it was really sweet, as you did not want to offend us. Thank you.

So, Sally, I finally felt that you were growing up. I still worried about your involvement with Sunrise Church, but it seemed to me that you were becoming less and less involved there. The worrying thing for me was that you also seemed to be a little lost in life. One of the things I loved to do was go to the coffee shop where you worked and say hi and order a coffee.

It somehow made me feel really proud when you told people that I was your mum and made a fuss of Lilly and Callum, if I had brought them with me. I loved to tell people where you worked and that you were my daughter. Everyone who had been to that shopping center knew who I was talking about because the coffee shop was at the entrance, and you have such a unique sense of style with hairstyles that are always so dramatic and eye catching, they recognized you instantly. Even as a little girl, you would tell me that when you grew up you were going to dye your hair black. I couldn't understand why you would want to change your hair color as you had beautiful naturally platinum blonde, straight, thick hair—every woman's dream! Not your dream, apparently, as from childhood you had plans for that hair of yours. Of course, you also made the best cup of coffee in the vicinity!

I think I loved acknowledging you in public because I kind of felt that when you were involved so heavily in the School of Signs and Wonders, it was almost as if you disowned us. When I met people from there, they would seem to be very surprised as though they assumed that you were in Australia by yourself. Of course, after you started to go to Sunrise Church, when we went to church or anywhere as a family, you never wanted to come with us.

It was during this time that your little brother Callum was diagnosed with Autistic Spectrum Disorder, in fact, not long before your twenty-first birthday. On the day of his diagnosis, I felt that my world had fallen apart and that I had lost a son and gained another child: a disabled child who was autistic. I truly think that at this time, I was going through a real period of intense grief for the loss of a child. I can't really explain it to someone who has not experienced that same thing. I felt like he had died, but that there was another boy running around the house in his body. On the outside, I looked the same and on the outside, he looked the same, but everything had changed. Your words were very comforting at this time. You said to me something along the lines of, "Mum, he is still the same Callum that he was before the diagnosis. It is just now his behavior has a label. He hasn't changed; it is your perception of him that has changed. He is still the same boy."

I took your words to heart and they were good to hear, but it still did not stop me grieving over what could have been. I know it is not very politically correct to speak like this, but it really was how I felt at the time. I was completely overwhelmed and felt so guilty that I had not picked it up sooner. As I started to research the disorder, I discovered that studies had proved that early intervention was the key to improving the chances for the individual to live a normal and independent life. I felt I had just about missed the boat; he was already five-and-a-half!

I spent weeks crying every time I was alone, but also was apt to burst into tears whenever anyone asked me about Callum. It took me months to actually process the diagnosis. Yes, now there was a name for a few of the things that I had been noticing about Callum, but it was not the name that I wanted. One of the things I remembered at this time was how he always seemed to have temper tantrums when I inadvertently changed something that had become a routine for him. Do you remember the time that we came into your work and you got him his customary order, which was banana bread? I can't remember what you did, probably cut it into quarters, and he became absolutely hysterical and would not eat it. It took me a while to figure out why he was hysterical and finally I realized that I usually cut it in half and then cut one of the halves into five fingers. At the time, I just thought he was being very difficult and naughty, but now I realize that any change in routine is very hard for people with autism and they have to be taught how to cope. So with the diagnosis, everything was slotting into place, but it was still a time of grief and trauma for me.

I had always thought he was a very brave boy, rarely crying when obviously hurt. Now I realized that he had a sensory processing disorder and also did not actually realize that he should cry when physically hurt. He could not dress himself and I had always assumed that it was because I had babied him a little, because he was the youngest, but now I was being told that he had gross motor deficiencies, fine motor deficiencies, low muscle tone and that he had dyspraxia, etc. In fact the list of things that were *wrong* with him nearly filled an A4 piece of paper. Of course, we knew that he often did not answer us when we spoke to him, but he could talk, so it never once entered my head that he had autism. I thought that autistic people were without speech. Now I know that some people with autism are non-verbal, but others speak; they just understand and use language in a completely different way.

We had taken him for a series of hearing tests after he suffered from a perforated eardrum and did not seem to be responding when we spoke to him. It appeared he did have a partial loss of hearing for a time. Then as the ear healed so did his hearing, but he still was not answering or following instructions. In fact, during the last hearing test, I remember the person administering the test had become quite impatient with both Callum and myself. He did not follow her instructions and I could not make him comply.

Really what this meant was that for the first year after Callum's diagnosis, I was totally focused on trying to:

> Come to terms with the diagnosis
>
> Learn about the diagnosis
>
> Apply for all the medical help I could get
>
> Seek out therapists to work with Callum
>
> Take him to numerous therapies every week
>
> Find a place for him in school
>
> Fight for him to get appropriate support in school
>
> Forgive myself for not realizing sooner that he needed help

This meant that I was consequently less focused on the rest of the family and for you, Sally, this was probably a good thing in some ways because it gave you time to be your own person. Perhaps it was also a bad thing because I was not aware that you were becoming increasingly unhappy with life in general and in particular, here in Australia. I had always been perturbed when you used to tell me that mentors you had at Sunrise Church wanted you to delve into your past hidden memories, the aim being to uncover incidents from your childhood that were stopping you from being free and thus preventing you from becoming a real Christian. I can't remember the exact words you used, but I remember I kept telling you that the Bible tells us to look forward not backward. I personally was worried that you would be induced into a state of remembering *false memories* as I had read research that suggested this was common. In fact, most of the time we had agreed not to talk about Sunrise Church because every time we did, we argued. You defended them to the hilt and would not hear a bad word about the leaders or any of their practices, teachings, or beliefs.

When we got permanent residency, I finally let go of trying to persuade you of the ills of Sunrise Church and decided to let you get on with your own life without my interference.

Was this the right thing? Only time will tell.

Love you dearly,

Mum

xxxx

LETTER 20

The Trip

Dear Sally,

So you are going on your world trip adventure. I am out of my mind with worry about the trip. I wish that you were going with a friend and not alone. I have tried to persuade you not to go, to wait, etc., but in the end, I can see that nothing I can say or do is going to stop you. You are on a mission and come hell or high water you are doing this thing. If I were you, I would wait until I had Australia citizenship before I went. If I were you, I would wait until I had saved up enough money for the trip. If I were you . . . but you know what? I am not you; you are you, and even though I am insanely anxious, I have to let go and realize that you are an adult and you make your own decisions.

Over the last few months, I have felt badgered over your constant requests for money for your trip. It has brought up every feeling of guilt and remorse over my parenting skills that I could ever imagine. The trip sounds amazing and I can see how it would appeal to you. I would love you to have the experience, but I simply cannot finance it. I cannot even lend you money that I do not have. It has deeply saddened me that I had to actually show you my bank statements before you would believe that we did not have a secret stash of money that I was keeping hidden from you. As you know, last year we bought the house we are now living in and the deposit took all our savings. I have even tried to explain to you that things are not going that well for us financially at the moment. I am unable to work, Leroy has spent time out of work, the therapies Callum needs and receives are exorbitantly priced, and generally, living in Sydney is very expensive.

Sometimes, I feel you are resentful to me for remarrying and I think that it hurts you to see the relationship that Leroy has with Lilly and Callum. Although not a perfect relationship, it is clear that he loves them overwhelmingly and maybe it is a reminder to you of the lack of relationship that you have with your own dad. Maybe this is why you put so much pressure on me sometimes, I don't know. I feel for you because I have had to be both mum and dad to you since your birth and sometimes, I feel that I have done neither very well. I would honestly love to be in the position to say yes to your request. I understand why you want the trip; personally, I would love to go to Canada and the United Kingdom to see family and friends that I miss so much.

In many ways, I think it will be great for you to get away from the influence of the church you have been involved with over the last few years. You know my opinion of that institution and its leaders. It is as though I have lost my daughter and they are responsible for your complete and utter brainwashing. They have abused and used your time and talents and when you crash, they will hang you out to dry. They seem to have fooled you into thinking that you are invincible and that you have special God-given powers. They have mesmerized you with their words of prophecy and knowledge. They have led you to believe that you can live a favored life and have encouraged you to believe that all your endeavors will have God's blessing and protection. You have been projected into a fantasy world. The special revelations and secret knowledge they purport to have are nothing short of a huge deception. Are they deluded or are they merely the deluders? Only God knows.

I am glad that you will be staying with people you know in Canada and that you will get a chance to spend time with Aunty Lina and Uncle Peter before they return to Kenya. Of course, you are really going to enjoy seeing all the friends you made when you spent the eight months in Canada with Aunty Lina. So I guess I am excited for you about that part of your trip. I also think it will be fantastic for you to get time to spend with Daniel in England. What a reunion that will be; how things have changed!

Sally, the parts I am most worried about are the trips to the United States and Europe. You will need a lot of money to survive and to travel there with no family, no funds, and on your own. What are you thinking of? I have a very strong feeling that I will be required to bail you out financially, but I am trying not to think about it or to project any outcomes. There is enough on my plate right now, right here in front of me, without me worrying what might be. The Bible is so right in saying that we should not worry about tomorrow. We should live each day as it comes—only God knows if we even have tomorrow. When I was in Al Anon, there was a saying I latched on to. It was "Do not let tomorrow's sorrow rob you of today's joy."

The years I spent in Al Anon taught me to live one day at a time. So often, I would spend my time worrying about whether or not your dad or Leroy would be drunk, and what the consequences of that would be, that I would not be able to enjoy the beautiful sunshine or a day at the park or a visit with friends or family. It got to the stage that even my days at work were consumed with fear for the future, the evening, the weekend. The whole time I would be worried about what awaited me on my return.

Since becoming a Christian, the maxim of living one day at a time has been re-enforced in my thinking. This day and this moment are all that we really have and we should lay hold of each day and live it to the full. Today is the day of salvation; no one, no matter how rich or powerful, can claim tomorrow, because it may never come for him or her. Of course, as a Christian, I want to live my life today in a way pleasing to God. I want to be a God pleaser, not a people pleaser. I also have to accept the things that are not in my power to change and I cannot change your decision to go on this trip so I will just have to let go and let you go.

I love you and I will pray for you every day.

Mum

xxxx

LETTER 21

Visa Denied

Dear Sally,

My stomach is churning again. I actually hate being proved right when it comes to things turning out badly. I am so sorry that you did not get the work visa that you were sure you would get in Canada. What will you do now? I have suggested to you that you return home, but you get very angry when I suggest it and have asked me not to suggest it again. Things are certainly not going as planned, but I have to remember that it is your life and not mine. I know deep inside that Leroy and I are going to have to bail you out financially and am feeling obligated to do so because you are my daughter and I love you. On the other hand, I feel that I need to allow you to face the consequences of your irrational actions. What does a mother do? Tough love is sometimes too hard. I guess because of all the tough love I have had to give Daniel and the accusations and guilt I have felt over decisions I made, I find this so hard.

The last few years have been so tough for me personally—moving to Australia, leaving everything I know yet again, and taking so long to feel any kind of normalcy—I fear I have put too much expectation on our relationship as mother and daughter. With having the rest of the family far away, I guess I wanted a special relationship with you. I always wanted you to be my friend and ally as you got older, but I now realize that we are not friends: we are mother and daughter. You are you and I am myself. We are very different and that is okay. Sorry if I placed an unreasonable expectation on our relationship. I have found it so hard to be on different sides from you in so many ways. It seems like every conversation has the potential to turn into a full-blown argument no matter what the topic.

The battle to get permanent residency here in Australia was long and very stressful. I believe it is nothing short of a miracle we got it considering my age (forty-nine) and the fact that everything depended on Leroy, his qualifications, and job prospects. It would have been so much easier if you had gone to a recognized college. However, we did get the residency, and for that, I thank God. When we moved here, I felt completely alone and bereft. Leroy had his job, Lilly had school, and I was just at home with Callum, a very active toddler who rarely slept! I never seemed to have any time, was constantly tired, often awake with Callum for hours during the night and then up all day, constantly in the car driving here, there, and everywhere. I had no friends and no family. After you arrived, you quickly got a job, started to go to church, and seemed to make lots of friends and have a very busy life. Very soon you were mobile and independent as we paid for you to have driving lessons and bought you your first car.

It did seem to me, though, that whatever we did, it was never enough for you. You constantly compared me to other parents and I of course, always came out as being, but a poor shadow of other people's parents. Every time I tried to give you advice, you rejected it. I remember trying to talk to you about the possibility that getting a working visa whilst in Canada would not be easy, but oh no, you had investigated it fully. What did I know? You would get the visa no problem. I do not like being proved right now that you do not have the visa. Sometimes, I wish you would just listen and not see me as the enemy, but rather as someone who loves and cares for you and does not want you to be in another country with little funds and no means of earning any to continue your trip.

Again, I am having to hand this over and let go of it, as it is not my life, but yours. The other aspect to all this is that Leroy is not your dad and has never really been able to step into the gap left by your own dad for you emotionally. In every way, Leroy has provided for you financially, but even though we have lived together as a family for twelve years, you have never felt like his daughter and he has never felt like your father. He is my husband and you are my daughter. Leroy has tried to provide you with guidance, but mostly you have rejected this guidance and just sought for acceptance. Being a woman myself, I know that teenage girls are very fragile whilst appearing to be indomitable. My own father never understood me or accepted me when I did not fit into his mould, but the fact that he was my biological father kept us speaking. In blended families, relationships are exponentially more complex. Stepparents, traditionally, are portrayed in a poor light. (From a young age we are fed stories of wicked stepparents. Think Cinderella and Hansel and Gretel.)

I cannot begin to imagine what it must be like to live with a stepfather, but I know that when I went to live with my Aunty Mae and Uncle Sam at the tender age of sixteen, I found it very awkward if I was alone with my Uncle. He was a very quiet man and often would not speak to me or acknowledge my presence. Then when my Aunt came in from work, he would talk to her about me and she would then approach me with any concerns that he might have. This left me feeling that he was spying on me, so that he could report to my Aunty. In actual fact, I now know that he was probably too shy or embarrassed to approach me personally and so left that up to my Aunty. I also now recognize what a supreme act of kindness it was for them to have me living in their house for two years. The house was small, a traditional three-bedroom semi on a council estate in the north of England. They were already a family of six, and I made seven. My four cousins were still at home and their ages ranged from fourteen to twenty-two. Although I loved them all, and got on with my aunty and cousins, I still felt like an outsider most of the time and never knew quite what to make of my uncle. On the other hand, he must have felt that his privacy had been completely breached now that he had his sixteen-year-old niece from Africa living under his roof. He could neither treat me as his daughter, nor as a stranger. What to do? What to say?

I know that Leroy has found it hard, even impossible, to be a dad to you, Sally, but I can only imagine how hard it has been for you. Your own dad has been absent for you, physically and emotionally, and since I married Leroy and had Lilly and Callum, you have been able to see Leroy's love in action for his own children. You have also been witness to our struggles with your brother Daniel, as he openly rebelled against us and against the school system. As for myself, I love you both dearly and my wish has always been that you would also love and respect each other. I have tried to compensate for the absence of your own father, but have to hold my hands up and say I have not always been able to do so successfully.

Leroy is a good man and has always tried to be honorable in his dealings with you, but he, too, has his limitations. As you now know, Leroy's symptoms that I thought were part of the process of recovering from alcoholism are in fact part of his persona that he was using alcohol to mask, i.e., his autistic tendencies. Since your little brother's diagnosis with autism, which, as you know, has completely rocked my world, Leroy has finally been able to put a name to his seemingly eccentric ways of thinking and acting. Callum's diagnosis has opened our eyes to Leroy's own personality. This may help to explain to you Leroy's struggles with social situations and small talk. He truly has no comprehension of the world of teenage girls, and perhaps you can see this even more clearly now, as Lilly is becoming a teenager and Leroy is completely perplexed and at a loss to know how to communicate on many occasions. His little girl is no longer; she has been replaced with a young lady—no longer a child, but not yet an adult—who is starting to question and be a separate person. Sometimes, she is moody and unresponsive; sometimes she is open and loving. Often, it is hard to know what to say.

The teenage years are fraught for both teenagers and their parents. For teenagers and stepparents, the road is even rockier. Many times, both of you have tried to bridge the gap, but never simultaneously. (I know that you are now no longer a teenager and are a young adult.) Both of you care for each other, but really only in the context of your respective relationships to me. What has all this got to do with the visa situation, you might ask? Well, it is just that it once again highlights the fact that Leroy is not your biological father. Logically, he will see no other solution to your dilemma other than that you should return home. He will not want to have to pay for your yearlong holiday. He will see this all very factually and no emotion will be involved. He will not understand that I will want to bail you out, although in the end, he will bail you out and will be left thinking that you only see him as a meal ticket. The way he will perceive it is that you do not want to listen to his guidance, but you want him to rescue you when you go against his guidance and things go wrong. In other words, he will feel used.

Rest assured, I know that this is not how you perceive him, but once again I feel like piggy in the middle. I am his advocate to you and your advocate to him. On the few occasions that I have abdicated this role, it has ended in disaster so I accept it, but it drains me emotionally. I am not able to tell you any of this at the moment because you are so far away and even if you were near, you are far away from me emotionally.

Over the last couple of months, I have had a small taste of what it is to be a live-in stepparent. This trip of ours to the United Kingdom, originally booked on the spur of a moment as Leroy's dad was only given two weeks to live, has ended up being a three-month trip and I now see that the real reason we are here is to assist Leo at this turning point in his life. I really have jumped in at the deep end, starting to be a live together stepparent with a twenty-four-your-old stepson who is an ex-heroin addict and is in the early days of coming off methadone. Being back here in the UK is amazing; we have been able to see friends and family and visit familiar places. It has truly felt to me like coming home. The most amazing part has been being able to reunite with Daniel and see the transformation in his life.

However, there have been times over the last couple of months when I have had glimpses of how Leroy must feel as he has tried to parent you, as I try to form a relationship with Leo. I have seen the bond between father and son that I am not a part of. I have seen Leroy's loyalties be divided between his son's wishes and my wishes. I have felt my privacy invaded and felt *watched.* I have noticed that my hackles rise more easily when Leo does not toe the line or when he disagrees, than if Lilly or Callum is being difficult. I do not like it when he has differing views to mine and expresses them forcefully. I find this very hard to admit as I have always expected Leroy to treat you and Daniel as if you were his own children and been disappointed when he has failed to do so. In many ways, he has treated you more favorably than his own children because he has expected less from you. This sounds like a paradox, but what I am trying to say is that in some ways, he has been less strict with you because you are not his own child. I can only really see this now as Lilly is in High School. You were allowed to get the bus or walk to school, but she is not. You were allowed to have a TV in your bedroom, but she is not. You were allowed to go out with friends in the evening, but she is not. He said to me at the very beginning of our marriage that he did not want to be a stepparent; he did not want to be the one to discipline you or make decisions about you. He was afraid that if he intervened in your lives, you would just turn around and swear at him, because he was not your real dad. He had seen this happen in the families of some of his friends and he wanted to avoid confrontation at all costs. He said, "I will look after you, and that will help you to look after your children."

Of course, life is not as simple as that and what has happened in reality is that his expectations of acceptable behavior, and mine, have differed. As a result, he has not always agreed with the way I have handled situations. So although he has left all the implementation of standards to me, in some cases, he has set the standards and I have had to enforce them; in others, I have set the standards and enforced them, but without backup. I have found in our present situation with Leo here with us that Leroy expects me to play a more active role with Leo than he ever has with you and Daniel. If I have a concern with Leo, he wants me to address it with him directly and not go through him. I empathize because this is how I have felt many times, but by the same token, I don't want to address it with Leo. I want Leroy to address it on my behalf! I do not want to be the *baddie.*

I know that Leroy must have had similar feelings of inadequacy and favoritism over the years. So I feel that God has given me this opportunity so I can have some empathy for Leroy and I hope that Leroy can now have some empathy with me.

When Leroy and I married in 1997, you were just ten, Daniel was eleven, and Leo, Leroy's son, was nearly twelve. Although Leo visited with his dad and us frequently over the first few years of our marriage, he did not live with us, and his visits rarely exceeded two weeks. This means that I did not really get the true feel of being a stepparent as in reality, I was only a holiday stepparent, which is very different. I know that the situations do not mirror each other as in reality—especially where you are concerned, Sally—I have been your only parent, whereas Leo lived with his own mum and visited with his dad, and so he didn't really need another mum, as you have needed a dad. If anything, Leo probably feels that he has missed out on a consistent father figure throughout his formative years. I wish all the dads out there would realize how important they are to their children. We all need a dad! I do think that if Leo had lived with us from the beginning, our relationship would be a lot closer than it is now, but I have not been able to put that to the test.

I know that Leroy feels he has been an inadequate father substitute and this makes him feel very guilty at times. Knowing what I know now, I accept that he has truly done the best he can. The only way he can really show that he cares is through financial assistance. Relationships are complex, even for us neurotypicals (those of us not on the autism spectrum), and this is no exception.

Back to the situation in hand, and the sick feeling in my stomach: I cannot see anything good coming out of this trip especially now that your visa has been denied, and you will not be able to earn any money legally in Canada, but I am trying not to worry about the long-term consequences for you and for us as a family. I am hoping that when you eventually get to the United Kingdom, you will be able to find work and will be able to recuperate financially before you return to Australia. I hope that you will be able to pay us back the money we have had to send to you, soon after your return. I love you through it all and am missing you, too! I so want Leroy to love you as much as I do and I want him to be proud of you, too. You do not have to prove anything to me. I am so proud of your tenacity and courage and determination. You are beautiful and kind and would not hurt a soul. I just want you to be happy and not to be deceived.

Love,

Mum

xxxx

LETTER 22

Trauma

Dear Sally,

On Mother's Day 2010, back in Australia, I ended the day being slightly irritated with you. Before our trip to the United Kingdom, we had sold the house we bought and started to rent another property nearby, which is where we were now living. Two days previously, it had been Callum's seventh birthday. We Skyped on his birthday, but you seemed a little weird and the Skype session was really short so I was expecting you to Skype again on Mother's Day. Although I always make a fuss of Leroy on Father's Day and get Lilly and Callum to make him cards and get him small gifts, he sometimes forgets to do the same for me. Daniel rarely remembers Mother's Day and if he does, it is the English Mother's Day, which is not the same date as the Australian Mother's Day. In some ways, it is a bit of a fake day, I feel. The real winners are the restaurants, florists, and confectioners. I know every time any of you have asked me what I wanted on Mother's Day, I have always said, "good behavior" or "peace in the house."

In reality, all I want from all my children and my husband is that they are kind to me and to each other and that they do what is expected without an argument. Of course, I would also love to escape from the kitchen for a day and find a clean car outside! But seriously, family harmony is the most important gift I could have. I guess society also puts the expectation on me that my children will actually remember that it is Mother's Day and care enough to do something about it! You, of all my children, have been the one who always remembers and gives me a card, which makes me feel special.

So on this morning, I did not have high expectations of the day, but I looked forward to seeing you on Skype. Callum's birthday had gone well. He had a swimming party and loved it. We opened all the presents at home afterwards, so the guests would not be offended if he didn't like their gift. He is not very good at hiding his feelings and although I have taught him to say, "Thank you for thinking of me," and to carefully put the offending gift down, instead of throwing it on the floor in disgust, his face cannot hide his true feelings.

I was glad you managed to say happy birthday to him and also that his cousins also wished him happy birthday. The only time he has ever seen them is when he was ten months old and of course, he can't remember that! As for this Mother's Day, I felt sad because I had not seen Daniel and you are away. My own mum is far away and I feel quite alone. For the past few years, you and I have always managed to have some special time on Mother's Day and it didn't happen today. At the end of the night and feeling slightly irritated with you, I decided to check my e-mail and noticed one from you. I opened it and that was the moment my life changed forever.

Oh my Lord and my God, how could this have happened to my sweet little baby girl? When I read what you had written, Sally, I instantly went into shock. I was cold and shaking and frozen to the spot.

I read the e-mail again.

I could not process what I was reading. I got up and reached the toilet just in time.

I called Leroy and showed him the e-mail. I started to cry. I wanted to book a flight straight away and rescue you. I wanted to feel you in my arms. I wanted to hug you tight and kiss you better.

I thanked God that you were alive. I felt like curling up into a ball, and hiding sobbing in a dark cupboard. I did not think that I could stand the pain of knowing.

I couldn't wait to see you on Skype. I was shaking. I felt completely and utterly useless. I felt abused. I wished it had been me and not you.

My first instinct was to start praying for you, which I did. As I was praying, some portions of the Bible came to my mind. I wanted to comfort you and the only way I could think of comforting you from so far away and through e-mail was to send you encouraging verses from the Bible that have sustained me since I became a Christian. I did not want to show you the pain I was feeling at that time because I sensed that you needed me to be strong. So I comforted myself with Psalm 23 and also sent it to you hoping that you would also find comfort there. I also sent you the Lord's Prayer because it is a model that Jesus gave to his disciples when they asked him how they should pray. In times of intense trauma and grief, we do not always have the words to express what we feel and sometimes actually words cannot begin to express what we feel, so at these times it can be helpful to use the words given to us by others, and what better words than those given by Jesus? He knows our pain; he suffered abuse, abandonment, and complete rejection from his family, his friends, his followers, his people, and God his Father. All this he suffered for us, for me and for you, Sally.

This thing that happened to you, Sally, is probably a parent's worst nightmare for their children. You lost more than the seven hours of your life that you cannot remember and you nearly lost your life. Being drugged, abducted, and violently raped repeatedly, is only one step up from death. I also lost my old daughter and gained a new one. Having this happen to your beloved child is something I would not wish on my worst enemy. Nothing will ever be the same again, for you and even for me. The thought still makes me want to curl up and die. Of course, I know that it is your pain and it is your trauma and it is your life, but I feel it for you. When I was younger, I did not understand why my parents hurt when something bad happened to me, but now I am a parent, I understand that parents hurt for their children. We have such a feeling of wanting to protect you.

Sally, when I found out what had happened to you, my hurt for you was intense and I have been grieving ever since for the loss of my old daughter. I know that you will never be the same person again, but I hope and pray that you will be a fuller, better, bigger person having survived that ordeal. Thank you, thank you, and thank you for trusting me enough to share this with me. I am honored

Remember I love you and always will. *You will recover!*

Mum

xxxx

LETTER 23

Trauma Revisited

Dear Sally,

Tomorrow is Callum's birthday and this year, Mother's Day is the following day. It is now one year since your trauma and what a year it has been.

I look back now and remember vividly how I felt and in fact how I still feel about the incident and I am perplexed by the actual response that I gave you at the time. It does not in any way reflect what I was feeling. It makes me wonder if I have hidden my true feelings for most of my life and I think that in many ways WYSIWYG (what you see is what you get) is definitely not the case with me. I have checked through all my e-mails at the time and found the one that I sent you in reply to you telling me what had happened. It is measured and almost emotionless; it shows love and gives encouragement, but gives no indication of how I was actually feeling at the time.

Once again, after this news, I was walking around this earth in a daze, continuing with life under the façade of normalcy, all the while feeling dead inside. If the truth were told, I am still walking around feeling dead inside. Mentally, I am unable to sustain the intensity of my feelings so I somehow seem able to shut off my functioning brain from the reality of what has happened and how it has impacted your life and also to a lesser extent the life of the family. Nothing really excites me anymore. If I got a letter and in it was check for $5,000,000 from a mysterious benefactor, I would be pleased as I would no longer have to worry money, but I would not be excited or jump about screaming with happiness. I would tell Leroy and I think he would jump about and immediately resign his job, but I would just bank the check and continue with daily life, one day at a time.

The first anniversary of your trauma has just passed and it seems hard to grasp that a year has gone by. Some really amazing things have happened in this year. Who would have believed that you, Daniel, and I would get to spend a week together in England, last July? That will remain for me as being one of the best weeks of my entire life. The circumstances that brought it about were intensely vile, but I was reminded of the verse in the Bible where Joseph is able to see that what his brothers intended for evil (selling him as a slave) God used for good (putting him in a position of power in Egypt so that he could prevent the starvation of his family). In the same way, I believe God brought some good into your evil-induced situation and allowed the three of us to be reconciled and be together physically for the first time in many years.

I hope that you can see and feel the love that I have for you as you have progressed through this ordeal and have started to rebuild your life. I also hope that you can see and feel the compassion that Leroy has felt for you by wiping clear the money you owed us and by giving you money to bridge the gap for you during the last few weeks you spent in Canada before continuing to England. I also hope you can see his compassion in putting aside past differences and providing a home for you for the past seven months where you have been able to live with us freely. It has not been easy for any of us and my heart goes out to you both constantly. In a way, Leroy has lost a wife over the last year, as my commitments to you and to Callum and Lilly have been so overwhelming that our marital relationship has had to take a back burner. I know he feels that he has become little more than a spare part, but in reality, I could not do any of this without him. He is the backbone of support in this family, both financially and spiritually. I admire him so much for being there for me in this difficult time. Many times, I know he wants us to spend time together as a couple, but all the time seems to get taken away as I am busy or feeling very distant as I try myself to come to terms with what has happened. As a man, I know it is very difficult for him; it has brought home to roost some of the fears he has for his own daughter, Lilly, your sister, and it has made him become even more protective over her. We have rarely let her out of our sight apart from when she is at school, but she is reaching an age now (twelve) where she should be able to do simple things like get the bus home from school instead of being picked up or go on a short errand to the local shops by herself. However, because of what has happened to you, Leroy is even more cautious than before and cannot contemplate these things.

I love you tirelessly and hope for you endlessly. I want you to be happy and fulfilled. I want you to come to that place where you are no longer looking back at events, but are looking forward to possibilities. I have no idea how you truly feel about what has happened, but I wish it had happened to me instead. Something has been stolen from you and you will not get those seven hours back, but you will recover your absolute sense of worth and dignity. In the meantime, the road is very rough and rocky and I am here to hold your hand and pull you up if you fall. I am so proud of you that you are pursuing the offender through the courts. You are one brave lady. I am praying for you constantly and imploring the God of Justice that justice will be done in this case. I know that ultimately justice will be served as the Bible teaches us that God will repay wrong doers. The Bible also teaches that we are to love our enemies and to pray for those that persecute us. I am finding that lesson hard to learn and to implement. I want to go up to that man and make him feel what he has done, especially to you, but also to our family.

The saddest and most scary thing about this whole affair is that I know you have been so close to taking your own life as a result of what has happened. I hope and pray that you never get that low again. There is a point in living and in carrying on; there is hope and a future. When you told me how close you were to committing suicide, down to the fact that you had actually planned your death and started the process one evening when the rest of the family was out, the pain of the thought hit me in that deep emotional place of my soul. For one instant, I contemplated the full horror of that situation and knew that it was more than I could bear. In fact, I still shudder at the thought. Many times I have felt low and many times I have wondered how I would be able to continue my life in circumstances that I have found unbearable, but every time I have continued and I believe every trial and difficulty have helped me to become a better person. At one time, I thought that my life was full of nothing, but hardship and disappointments and that everyone else around me had good luck, good times, and perfect families. As I get older, I find that life is tough for all of us and the difference really is in attitude—it is in the mind. I try to look for the good in every situation, however bad. I thank God every day that I wake up in a comfy bed, have food in the cupboard to give my family, and have a roof over my head. My family has clothes to wear and most importantly, we have each other.

I know that this is no consolation to you at this time. My heart bleeds that I have not been able to protect you from the evil that happened.

You and I have been able to sit down and accept that had this not happened, we would not have had this opportunity to spend so much time together and would not have grown as close as we have. This is time that we should cherish as I am confident that once you are back on your feet again and living your own life to the full, we will not be able to spend so much time together. It is as if your life has been put on hold and at this time, I am here to be with you during that pause. Of course, the fact that you broke two bones in your foot one month after returning home from your trip, were virtually immobile for four months, and are still recovering physically has really meant you have had to stop and be still. This has given you time to reassess your life and I hope it has helped you to see what is important and what is not. I know that it has helped you to determine who your real friends are, as they stick by you in adversity, and which of your friends are only "good times" friends.

Your adversity and my reaction to it have also been teaching me a few things about myself. I have lost part of myself and have come to realize how imperfect a person I really am. I am not as forgiving and loving as I thought and I am relying entirely on God to get me through each and every day. I am learning that sometimes less is more and that the less I say about any given topic the better. I want to talk to you about what happened and how the court case is progressing, but I am learning that I must wait for you to tell me. At the same time, I continue to find your behavior infuriating and annoying at times and of course, the moment those feelings appear, I feel guilty because of what has happened to you. I hate it, especially when you are careless with your safety or when you take out your feelings on me.

I want to show you what to do and how to get better, but I have to step back and allow you to be in control of your choices regarding your own recovery and also allow you to respond to the circumstances of your own life. I have to trust God that he will hear my prayers and draw you closer to him for full healing. I have come to realize that I can be a bit of a control freak; I want everything to run smoothly *my way!*

It is funny how the practicalities of home life can undo all the high and lofty ideas you have about yourself. There is nothing like a sink full of dirty dishes to bring out the worst in me, unless it is people complaining about a lack of food when the fridge and cupboards are full of food. I hate sharing a kitchen and I never knew I was like that! So I find myself boiling up with resentment and anger over stupid insignificant things and then covering over my feelings because I feel I shouldn't have them. Also, I am always conscious how hard the situation is for Leroy and how he finds any sort of confrontation hard to handle. I know that he wants to protect me from any sort of confrontation, but that he also misinterprets normal disagreements and heated discussions as being something more than they are. You and I are learning that we are very different. We hold differing views on most topics, but we are also learning that that is okay. We can agree to disagree and still love and respect each other. Leroy, on the other hand, seems to see disagreement as a rejection of principles and respect. It is hard enough for adult children to go back and live with their parents, never mind doing it in a situation such as ours.

Since you opened up to me and told me how suicidal you have been feeling, it has made me step back a little. I am trying very hard not to be judgmental and to allow you to be you within the boundaries that living in community brings. I have noticed how respectful you are of our views on loud music and how you use headphones. I have noticed how respectful you have become over watching TV. (You now turn it off or over immediately you are asked to do so.) You are now more understanding of Callum and his autism and understanding of Leroy's need for quiet in the house. You have made many attempts to get on with Lilly and that is beginning to pay off. You may not be able to see that you are making any recovery, but you are. You are no longer biting my head off every time I speak to you. You are beginning to have a plan of action and are starting to be up during the day and in bed during the night. There is a light at the end of the tunnel.

In my life, I have come to realize that we are not responsible for the way other people treat us, but we are responsible for the way we treat other people. What I mean to say is we cannot control the actions of another person. The only actions and thoughts we can control are our own. So this, in fact, makes us free in regard to certain situations in our life. If we were not in control, we are not responsible and therefore, there is no guilt attached. Our own responses to others and how we react to our circumstances are within our control and these are the actions we want to ensure are true to who we are. We do not want to have any regrets about them. I have come to understand that crimes such as rape are not actually primarily sexual; they are in fact about control and power. One person subdues another and forces that person to do something they do not want to do. When date-rape drugs are used, the victim is not even aware of what is happening and so is not even able to make any decision as to whether it is safe to protest or not. This is what happened to you and you should in no way feel any responsibility for what happened that night and I am sure that you do not.

Have I said how proud I am that you are taking this through the courts? You have my total support and backing. Whatever the outcome, you are doing the right thing and you are taking control over what happened. And my darling, even if it gets too much and you decide to drop charges before the actual trial, I will still be proud of you for taking it as far as you have. In the end, I believe justice will be served, as I believe that God will execute justice either in this life or the next. The human courts may not execute justice all the time, but the offenders never escape God's judgment.

I know that the times when I was raped were very different. For me, it was more a case of being deceived and manipulated. I was aware of what was happening, but at the same time, I didn't actually know what was happening. It seems silly to me now that I did not know, but I was truly deceived. Of course, by the time I did realize that I had had sex— the real deal—I found it too difficult to protest successfully. I protested, but was then manipulated into having sex either by physical force or by emotional bribes. I know that you feel my sorrow at what has happened to you is exasperated by the fact that I never did anything about what happened to me. In the end, I basically ran away from the situation and perhaps it is as you say and I am only really facing the facts of what happened to me now, as I face what has happened to you. Who knows?

Recently I saw a book compiled by Elton John, where he had asked a collection of celebrities to write a letter to their sixteen-year-old self. Well, if I could write a letter to my seventeen-year-old self before the unwanted sex and the unwanted abortion, I would write;

> Having a boyfriend is not important.
>
> Forget the French homework; you are going to get a crap mark anyway. Instead, do some research, and find out exactly what sex is so that you are not deceived.
>
> Talk to your friends and family and tell them what is happening in your life.
>
> Listen to the advice of trusted, older people; they know what they are talking about!
>
> Trust God and pray every day. Read your Bible and truly believe what it says.
>
> Be assertive, but not aggressive and stand up for what you believe in.

Of course, I would also write, *do not go out with Colin,* but if I had followed all the above, I wouldn't have gone out with Colin, would I?

The point I am trying to make, my dear Sally, is that there are some situations that with hindsight could have been avoided, but we are not gifted with hindsight so we learn as we go. I feel that the pregnancy that ensued from my relationship with Colin and the subsequent abortion have affected my whole life and no doubt what happened to you will affect your whole life, but not all for the bad. Because I had a teenage pregnancy, my cousin was able to come to me when she got pregnant and know that I would not judge her. At the time, she didn't know what to do and I advised her strongly not to have an abortion. The result is her beautiful son who is getting married this year. Also in the case of being a victim of a crime, we are not the guilty ones—the perpetrators are.

I know that you have told me that you have been advised that you need to feel that you are back in control of your life and therefore I must not speak to you about the rape unless you bring it up. This enables you to be in control of when you talk about what happened, and who gets to know about it. I understand this and before you read this letter, I will tell you that it makes reference to what happened so that you are in control of when you read it.

There is so much as a mum that I want to say to you that I don't end up saying when we are speaking because the practicalities of life take over and also because you have placed a restriction on me regarding the subjects I can talk about. Talking has been difficult lately. When I talk about other members of the family, you chastise me and say that that is all I ever talk about and you don't want to know about others. When I talk about my life or my feelings, you say that you are not interested in what I have to say because you have too much to deal with yourself. When I talk about you and your life, you say it is none of my business and I should stop interfering. When I don't talk, you ask me what is wrong and say that I am rude and uncaring. Rarely, we get those moments when you feel like talking and I am able to listen without reproach or interruption and they are like rays of sunlight bursting through an otherwise dark sky.

Thank you so much for the dinner you cooked for this Mother's Day. I can't tell you how good it was to get home from church and find such a beautifully cooked meal all ready and waiting. One day when you are a mum, you will realize that acts of service are very much appreciated by mums as we spend so much of our lives in acts of service to our families. I loved the thought that you put into the presents and dessert at

The Chocolate Restaurant with you and Lilly was so special. A year on, there is still much pain, some of it unspeakable, but this day was much happier than last year. I hope that we have many more to celebrate together.

Love,

Mum

xxxx

LETTER 24

Good News, Visas, Visits, and Stuff

Dear Daniel,

Well, how our lives have changed. I got up this morning and knocked on your bedroom door to tell you that it was 8:30 and I was off taking Lilly and Callum to school. So here you are at twenty-five years old finally at home again with us and in Australia. In a couple of weeks, it will be your twenty-sixth birthday and I am so excited that we will be able to celebrate it with you. Christmas and New Year were amazing. I don't think you will ever know how much it means to me that you and Leo were with us for those times. Of course, it is not the same as having you home as a teenager, and there is still a lot of hurt there on both sides, but the fact that you are here and we are able to hug and tell each other that we love each other despite all that has gone on is nothing short of a miracle. I know that in another month you will be on your way back to the United Kingdom and the visit will seem like a dream, but I am trying to savor every moment. This may be the only time that you visit here and is probably the only time you will visit with us for such an extended period.

Of course, none of this could have happened without something drastic happening in your life. Where do I begin?

It is now more than five years since that change occurred in your life and I look back in amazement at the events at that time. Although our first year here had been very traumatic, we had decided to stay on and apply for permanent residency. I had written to you to tell you that we were not coming back. I think that this may have been one of the things that prompted your deepening despair.

Then one day, I had an e-mail from you and it was really messed up. The spelling was poor and sentences were disjointed, but the message was, "My life is not worth living."

I felt so hopeless; what could I do? I knew that your life was not worth living. I had spent so many sleepless nights praying for you in your dreadful situation. Now here I was in Australia and too far away to do anything else but pray. I phoned my cousin Carol and she had not seen you for a long time. My prayers for you intensified. I really felt that this would be a turning point in your life, but I did not know whether it would be for the good or whether you would go deeper into a world of crime, prison, or maybe even suicide.

Then I had a phone-call from Carol saying that you had rung her and that she had invited you over for dinner the following Sunday. She was going to ask you to go to church. Somehow I just knew that this was going to be the beginning of something good. I had a good feeling in the pit of my stomach about you for the first time in years. I did not hear from her until a few days after your visit, but even before she rang, I knew that it would be good news. By the time she rang, you had had the visit and you had made a commitment to leave your old life behind and had become a Christian. What was also amazing was that you were already in a Christian Rehab Centre and had left your old neighborhood. For years I had tried to get you into a rehab and either they were too expensive or you would not agree to go. Carol told me that I would not be able to communicate with you for at least a month and that after that communication would be very limited. I know that rehabs operate in this way to give the person a chance to get their life in order without the distraction of past relationships, but I found it to be very frustrating as all I wanted to do was jump for joy and speak to you on the phone. In fact, for about two or three weeks after the news, I was walking on air. I was so overwhelmed by God's goodness and by your change of heart and direction that I was in an elated state. It must have showed on my face because parents at the school where Lilly was going were asking me what had happened, and some told me that my face was literally glowing. When I explained to them why I was so happy, some of them were overcome with emotion themselves and said things like, "Oh, the hairs on my neck are standing up!" or "That is so wonderful it has given me goose-bumps all over!"

Daniel, from the moment of your conversion to this, it has been as though a heavy burden was lifted from my shoulders.

Eventually, a couple of months later, we spoke and from that moment I started working on trying to get you to apply for a visa to visit us here in Australia. I was hoping to get you out here for your twenty-first birthday, but when I made enquiries to immigration consultants, they said there was no chance of you getting a visa until you had a five-year gap from your last offence. Believe me, when I heard that news, I felt like someone had kicked me in the stomach. Leroy will tell you that I bent over double and could not breathe. My pain was actually physical. After that subsided, I could not stop crying for days. It seemed like such a slap in the face from God.

Through it, I learned that good things are worth waiting for and began to accept that my timing is definitely not always God's timing. Our relationship was so broken and dysfunctional that in retrospect, it has probably been a good thing that we have had to wait to spend such a concentrated time together.

To have you here with us now is like a dream come true. I will remember the last few months for the rest of my life. Of course, I am not pretending that we have all carried on as if nothing ever happened, but this has certainly been a time where we have had a chance to get to know each other again. Our two trips to the United Kingdom in 2009 and 2011 started the reconciliation process. I can't even describe to you how I felt when I saw you for the first time after four years and you were standing outside your accommodation at the Bible College in York. My son at Bible College: it was unreal. It was fantastic, but what was even better was being able to put my arms around my son and give him a hug and tell him I loved him and not have him push me away. Those visits started the process of healing, but I know there is still some way to go even now. I remember going out with you one day for the whole day in Wales and we spent most of the time just talking about the past. You asked me about various times in your life that you said you could not remember clearly because your brain was a bit fuzzy with taking drugs. You could not remember sequences of events especially relating to when I kicked you out the first time. We were able to talk openly and honestly and were able to speak forgiveness to each other. At the end, I was crying and I remember you saying that I should not cry and we agreed that from then on, we should only look forward and not backward. I remember thinking at the time that sometimes it is not as simple as that because our past can creep up on us unexpectedly, but I agree that we need to focus on looking forward.

Part of the healing was you making this trip over to Australia. You may never comprehend how huge this was for me. It seemed that the time was never going to be right. When you really wanted to come (in the first year after you became a Christian) it was not possible and then when it became possible, it seemed that you did not want to come because of other things going on in your life. So when you came, I was trying just to let you be you and to get to know you again. Of course, I had a tendency to treat you as a sixteen-year-old because that is how old you were when you finally left home, but I gradually got the message that you were nearly twenty-six and a lot had happened in your life since then. You were a man. To me, though, you were still my boy and I still felt the way I did when you were a newborn baby, I wanted to show you off to the whole world. I wanted to shout to the world, "This is my son; he was lost, but now is found." I am not sure you will ever understand this. Maybe one day if you ever have the privilege of being a parent yourself, you will.

In the meantime, old hurts still haunted me from time to time and I am sure that they haunted you, too. You felt rejected and so it seemed to me that sometimes you wanted to keep your distance from me and the rest of your family on my side. You have so long lived with your peers and contemporaries that you seemed to find family life, which can be very mundane especially with younger siblings, boring. You wanted to be apart from us and make your own friendships here in Australia. You didn't want to be big brother and son; you just wanted to be you. I understood this, but sometimes it hurt and I was reminded of when you refused to call me *Mum,* only used my first name, and would not walk down the street with me. You knew this because we spoke about it. So I guess what I am saying is pretty much in line with the idea that broken relationships are not magically fixed in a day. I am so grateful for those months where we had time to start working on our mother/son relationship. It was a joy to get to know you again and to hear what other people have to say about you. I was particularly impressed with the way that you were respectful of Leroy and conformed to the rules of our house, which at times must have been very hard for you. You are an amazing young man and your life is a testimony of what God can do with one messed up boy. May he continue to work in each of our lives.

In some ways, you are more like me than you might think. I felt very abandoned by my parents at many stages in my life, particularly when I fell pregnant at seventeen, but also each time I was sent to boarding school or left in a hostel. I was also completely without any close family from the age of sixteen. At that age, my parents were in Africa and my sister was in Canada. From the age of eighteen, I had to fend for myself completely and although I had somewhere to live during term time when I attended teacher-training college, I had nowhere to go during the holidays and so used to look after flats for other students who had gone home. I had nowhere to go to take my washing, sleep or get a few free meals and always had to find work so that I could eat. This was good in that it taught me to fend for myself and not to rely on others to support me, but it also made me hard and bitter. I resented that others seemed to have it easier than I did and I kept a grudge against my parents for their failings.

I can truly say that when I became a Christian, I was healed of these bitter feelings, but it was not immediate. On the day after I became a Christian, I rang my mum to tell her the news, but I almost said it in passing even though I knew that it was what she had wanted to hear for years. I told my sister in much the same way. It was hard giving them joy when I had felt so bitter for so long. It was too late for me to reconcile with my dad, as he was dead, but I have now been able to truly reconcile with my mum and that has been wonderful. As I get older, I realize that no one is a perfect parent and that we all make mistakes. I know that my parents loved me. I know that whatever their reasons, they always felt that they were making decisions for my benefit. I still don't agree with some of those decisions, but have been able to let go. I hope that one day you will be able to completely let go of any feelings of resentment and bitterness that you might have over my failings as your parent. I love you and always have.

Love,

Mum

xxxx

P.S. Reading over this last letter, I realize that I left out a lot of *good stuff.* So here we go. These are my best memories of you in the last year in the United Kingdom when we visited, Italy on the holiday, and here in Australia: The tanning, the work outs, walking the dog the first night you got to Australia and getting lost, the rapping in your room, the bursting out in song in the kitchen, the Bible reading, having a conversation with you and then realizing you haven't heard a thing because your headphones were in, or thinking you were talking to me and realizing that you were in fact on Skype with a friend in the United Kingdom, New Year's Eve at the Outlook, the showers, the showers, did I mention the showers? The obsession with brushing your teeth, your gleaming white T-shirts, socks and pumps and last, but not least the caps for every occasion.

The special times were when we were able to have a coffee together, or went to the cinema or for some time out. I loved both our day out alone together and the time in New Zealand when you joined us for a family holiday and took part in the same activities as us. You showed me that you are a very independent person who likes to do things his way and I admire your ability to go out there and make friends.

Thank you for introducing Lilly to the Youth Group at the local church and encouraging her to attend.

I was also impressed by your zeal for telling people about Jesus and that you shared your faith with anyone who would care to listen. (The man outside the toilets at Castle Towers with a cross tattoo on his hand being a case in point.)

You changed from the boy who wouldn't do anything to the man that does all he is asked. So, for all your washing up, vacuuming, mopping, shopping, and gardening: thank you. Thank you also that you followed our rules in the house without complaint; this was the most obvious sign of a transformed life.

One of the best nights in my life was when I went to hear you do a gig at a Starbucks in Manchester. You performed a rap that you had written, which was about the transformation in your life, but it was not that, that touched my heart. It was the fact that you told everyone that your mum was in the audience and you said publically that you loved me. You will never, never know how much that public acknowledgement of me as your mum meant to me and it was why I broke down in tears.

I hope that your stay here in Australia was all that you hoped it would be and I pray that you remain, *Steadfast, immovable, always abounding in the work of the Lord, knowing that your toil is not in vain in the Lord. 1Cor 15v58.*

I can't wait to see what happens next in your life and I hope that it includes a wife who has your passion for serving God.

Mum

xxxx

3

To My Stepson—Leo

A Ready-Made Son

Well, Leo,

It feels a little strange writing you this letter. I feel like a bit of a fraud because you are not my birth child. I am not even sure how you will feel reading it. You are indeed someone else's son and you have a mother of your own, whom you love dearly, but you are also my son, my stepson. When I married your father in 1997, you were part of the deal. I had my two children and he had you, only it was different because they lived with me whilst you lived with your mother. She is the one who has raised you and was there with you during all your formative years. Not only did you not live with us, but also, we did not live nearby and visitation was usually during the school holidays and involved travelling from Scotland to firstly London and then to Stoke-on-Trent.

Those early years of my marriage to your dad were very difficult and that is an understatement. Your dad was still drinking and in fact the first year of our marriage was his worst year of his drinking. Coupled with that, I got a new job with extra responsibilities and the school was expecting me to turn a department around in time for an OFSTED (Office for Standards in Education) inspection. Just to complicate matters even further, I fell pregnant not long after your dad and I were married, so when we moved back to Stoke, I started my new job at nearly six months pregnant. Of course, you know all this, but what you do not know is that when your dad and I got married, I was very naïve about how it would all work out. You seemed to get on okay with Daniel and

Sally and I really admired the fact that your dad paid maintenance to your mum and that he regularly had you for visits and was always buying you things. He clearly loved you a great deal and was always concerned about your welfare. This was in contrast with what I perceived to be the attitude of Daniel and Sally's dad.

Your dad and I had not really talked through how everything would work out with you children. We had not talked about finances, who would pay for what, nor had we talked about discipline or how we would treat all of you fairly. At the beginning, we were almost like two partial families living together. It was assumed that I would pay for everything for Daniel and Sally and that your dad would pay for you. It soon became apparent that you had better clothes and better possessions than Daniel and Sally. Also, because you did not live with your dad, he obviously wanted to treat you and make every visit special, so he tended to buy you expensive gifts when you visited and take you on expensive trips. This continued after your dad and I met and caused Daniel and Sally to feel jealous, as I could not afford to do the same for them and it also made me feel inadequate. Financially, I was still operating as a single parent, paying the mortgage on two properties (London and Stoke), paying for childcare whilst I worked, and receiving no financial help from their father. On the contrary, your dad had a lot of disposable cash. He bought the food from time to time, paid for some furniture, family outings, and a trip to the Lake District, but initially left all the bills to me. Just after your dad and I met, he took you on a trip to Disneyland Paris, which Daniel and Sally accepted, as at that time your dad and I were not married. After we married, he continued to be extravagant with you. I remember that he bought you a pool table and then travelled up to Scotland to install it in your grandma's attic. You tell me now that it was with money he had put into a savings account for you, but you see, Leo, I never had enough money to put into a savings account for Daniel and Sally so it still seemed extravagant.

After we moved back to Stoke, my finances were temporarily better as I sold the flat in London so only had one mortgage to pay, but the money I made only paid off some of my debts. I found it very hard to talk to your dad about money and indeed any debts I had before we met were not his responsibility. It was just that we did not really start off on an even footing and at that time we kept our finances separate. All of the money I earned went on bills and housekeeping and your dad's just seemed to go on his personal expenses, treats, and of course, alcohol. He still seemed to have a lodger mentality and because we had not discussed it before we got married, and because his drinking had become so obsessive, it was not easy for me to "spoil" his sober times by talking about finances. (I was just relieved he was not drinking.)

I continued to keep silent. More and more, I was wondering what I had gotten myself into. It all came to a head when he booked a trip to Disneyland Florida for you, his brother Andreas, and himself. Daniel and Sally were very upset and I had to sit down and explain to them that I simply could not afford to pay for them to go. I was heavily pregnant at the time and would not have been able to go anyway. At the time, I had too much else to worry about to consider talking about finances as your dad had been on a six-week drinking binge since the funeral of your great-grandmother. I was quite simply at my wits end: new marriage, new stepson and new job, pregnant at forty and having been advised by the medical profession that my baby would be Down's syndrome. I guess I was not really the ideal mum, never mind stepmum!

I really could not see how the marriage was going to last and was barely holding it together for my own kids. Then the trip to Florida happened. I had been so worried about your dad that I had managed to persuade him to go to AA before he left for the trip. Actually, he must have really wanted to go, as I could never have persuaded him to do anything he didn't want to do! I know now he was really desperate, but then it just seemed to me that he had a self-destruct button that he was happily pressing. He managed to come off his bender and was dry for a day or two before he was due to fly (or so I thought).

When I took you to the airport, he was very anxious to get through to the departure lounge and I guess at that point I realized that his only desire was to get to the bar on the other side. The rest is history with your dad nearly drinking himself to death on that holiday, which must have been nothing short of a nightmare for you. Fortunately, your Uncle Andreas was with you and I imagine he looked after you on that trip because from all accounts, your dad was too busy drinking.

Of course, you were far more aware than I of your dad's drinking problem, as you had known him a lot longer. You had also been with him during drinking sessions on many occasions. This particular binge has a different ending as it culminated in your dad being taken by ambulance to Wythenshawe Hospital. He reached his rock bottom on that trip, but it was enough to put him on the road to recovery, and as you and I know, he hasn't had a drink since. I believe that he nearly died on the plane trip back from Florida and am thankful to God that he did not. He went through a *de-tox* at the hospital and came home a week later.

On that day, I brought you and Andreas home with me and later took you to the station where you got a train back to Scotland. I don't really know what you thought about that holiday or what effect, if any, it had on you. Sally has told me since that Daniel and she felt very much like the second-class children at that time and both of them would have loved to go. Of course, now that they know the truth about what it was like, they are glad that they didn't. I guess the point I am trying to make is that I did not know what you thought then and I also don't really know what you think now. It is only very recently that I have discovered the story behind your trip to Florida and I now understand why your dad took you and Andreas and did not think to include Daniel, Sally, or myself.

You shared the details behind this trip recently as part of your life's story at a church here in Australia. It appears that some time before I met your dad, he had been drinking heavily one night whilst visiting you in Scotland, but decided to take you and your uncle (his brother) out to get some videos for you to watch and also to get some more booze for himself (of course!). On that fateful day, he was stopped by police, given a breathalyzer test, found to be over the limit, and taken to the police station. I could identify completely with your description of what followed. You described waiting for your dad to come back with your uncle in your grandma's house. Andreas had been so scared of how your dad would be that he had gone out and bought the booze that your dad was going out to buy, put it in the fridge and you were just sitting quietly in a corner playing with some Lego bricks. When your dad returned, you talk about just looking at his face and knowing that trouble was about to blow. You then explained the feeling you get when you know that someone is really angry and you are afraid that their anger will be directed at you, so you just sit as quietly as you possibly can, hoping they won't even notice you are there. The room goes very quiet and you can feel the tension in the air. I know that feeling, Leo, because it is the feeling that I have felt many times and it is the feeling that families of alcoholics all feel at one time or another. Your stomach begins to churn and you want the ground to swallow you up. You would rather be anywhere else in the world and you just want it to be over and everything to be okay again.

You explained that Andreas tried to calm your dad by telling him that you had been to the off-license, bought him the beers he was after and put them in the fridge. Your dad then turned to you and said, "What are you laughing at?"

Of course, you weren't laughing—just scared and probably had a very nervous look on your face. When you denied laughing, your dad strode over to where you were and kicked the Lego you were playing with all over the room, completely trashing it. You were so upset that you ran out of the house and back to your mother's house.

The next day, after sobering up a little, your dad was full of remorse and he went to your mother's house to see you and told you that to compensate for what he had done, he would give you anything you asked for. Not to miss the opportunity of a lifetime, you asked for a trip to Disneyland Florida, with your Uncle Andreas to come along. Your dad then promised to take you both on the trip. This is the trip that you went on a year after I married your dad. I had no idea at the time why he was taking you other than you had asked to go and he had made a promise to take you. Of course, your dad did not tell me the full story as he would have felt very ashamed of his behavior, but I also understand now that he was fulfilling an obligation to you and so did not think how it would look to his new wife and stepchildren.

The relationship that I have with you is different from the one I have with the other children, but in one way we are closer in that we both love your dad and knew him in his drinking days. To Daniel and Sally, your dad is their stepdad; they are not in it as deep as we are. To Lilly and Callum, your dad is their dad, but they have never known him to take a drink so have been blessed with a sober dad. Thank God they have never known the pain of watching someone drink themselves to destruction, but they have also never known him as the life and soul of the party, the visionary, the optimist. In fact, the relationships I have with each of you are different from the others and that is because you are all different, but there is something about being the natural mother that overrides everything else. I am sure that your own mother feels the same about you. The relationship I have with you is because I am married to your dad and it is also because I am married to your dad and love him that I love you, too, as you are part of him. You are also the brother of our two children together, Lilly and Callum, so you share a blood relationship with them. You are truly part of our family even though our family is not your whole family.

Recently, I have tried to come to terms with the fact that I married two alcoholics, more especially that I married your dad after knowing the despair of living with an alcoholic. Truthfully, I did not know he was an alcoholic when I married him, and he did not drink in the same way as Daniel and Sally's dad who was an *everyday* drinker. Your dad could go days, weeks and even a couple of months without a drink, but then when he drank, he just did not stop. He managed to hide much of his drinking from Daniel and Sally. They were aware he drank; I am not sure that they realized what a problem it was. He was not really a violent drunk and pretty much kept himself to himself when drinking, confining himself to the bedroom. In the meantime, they just got on with life as normal. Your dad had asked me not to tell them when he went to AA or that he had a drink problem. I respected his wishes although now, I wish I had told the truth to them, as it caused so many more problems later on. I could not be honest with them about why he was in hospital or where he went when he continued to go to AA after he was discharged and I did not like being deceitful.

You continued to visit us from time to time in Stoke after Lilly was born and it always seemed to be me that was looking after you, as your dad was always working and I was the one at home, either on maternity leave or school holidays. This I found quite tough and sometimes wished that your dad would be the one to supervise your visits more closely. You seemed to get on quite well with Daniel and Sally, but were allowed to do things that I had never allowed them to do so I found it hard to maintain my standards. One example was that you were allowed to watch films of any rating and also your dad did not mind you swearing and using expletives. On the other hand, you were always very polite to me and rarely openly defiant. I began to understand a little of how your dad must have felt, being a stepparent to Daniel and Sally. He was really hands off, but always seemed to notice if they were disobedient or argumentative and came to me to ask me to do something about it. He didn't understand how I would not notice some of the things they did wrong, but it was the same with me. Your dad seemed blind when you disobeyed some of his rules (for example, not eating in the living room), but I would notice. I always felt like I was the one telling you off. Parenting sure is a complicated thing and being a stepparent is even more complicated. In disputes, you always instinctively believe your own child over your stepchild, even though you fight in your head to be fair. It is just a fact of life. Maybe it would be different in different circumstances, for example, if your stepchild lived with you from the beginning of your marriage or if they were very young when you became the stepparent or if the real mother/father was deceased, but that was not the case with us.

I don't feel like I met your emotional needs in any way and I am sorry that I was not more relevant in your upbringing, I really did not want to step on your own mother's toes as she is the one that brought you up. She is the one who was there for you when you were growing up. I am not a very confident person and never wanted anything to do with your own mum. As far as I was concerned, that was another part of your life and was really none of my business. The only things I knew about your mother were the things that your dad had confided in me when we first met, or things that you, Daniel or Sally told me. I know that after Daniel stayed with you for a couple of weeks when you were both thirteen that he came back with a very negative view of your dad and it seemed to me that he had learned things about him from the both of you, which set him against his stepdad. However, such is life. I wished I had not allowed him to visit with you and your mum, but I can't change the fact that I did. I know that on this visit you both smoked cannabis, but I suspect that he would have gone down that route anyway. I also know that it is hard to bring up children single-handedly, which is what your mum has largely had to do, and which I have also had to do with my older children. We all make mistakes and wish we had done things differently. I was only in charge of you when you were with us and really what I did was provide for your physical needs, food, shelter, and activities.

Looking back, some would say that I focused too much on Lilly and her eczema and basically took my eye off the ball with you, Daniel, and Sally. As long as you were reasonably well behaved and out of my hair, I did not really interfere. I had post-natal depression after having Lilly, and this was compounded with living with your dad who was a recovering alcoholic and who was coming to terms with the reality of life without his crutch—alcohol. The genial father figure, who frequently bought sweet treats for you kids from the off-license when he went to buy his poison and who then retreated to his world of make believe and let the world go by, was now in that world of crying babies and turbulent preteens. Living with your dad as a drinking alcoholic was not easy as his life was ruled by alcohol. He was totally unreliable and I was basically watching him kill himself. Living with him after he sobered up was also not easy as we both had huge adjustments to make.

To this day, it makes me shudder when I hear the sound of a can top being popped open as it brings back the memories of hearing beer can tops being popped open all though the night through the worst of your dad's drinking. However, I cannot lie and say that it was bad all the time. I fell in love with your dad when he was a drinking alcoholic (even though I did not know it at the time). He was full of optimism and had great plans. He certainly was not boring. He was always thinking of things to do and places to go and had a great spirit of adventure. In fact, I had never met anyone who made me feel the way he did and still does. He always defended me to others and would stand up for me in a way that no one else had ever done. He seemed to believe in me.

Conversely, living with him as a recovering alcoholic was no picnic, as he had lost his crutch and he required a silent or giggling baby and perfectly behaved children. He would not let any of you take Lilly out for a walk in her pram or pick her up. It seemed I was the only person he trusted with Lilly. I had to do everything and he would not allow babysitters. He didn't really even trust me with her and was constantly ringing me up from work to make sure that she was safe. He himself was scared of being left alone in the house with her, so I felt completely trapped and could not even take you guys out to the park without taking her with me. If Lilly started crying, I had to get her quiet or he would leave the house with his hands over his ears. Of course, she had eczema so cried quite often as it hurt and because I did not want your dad to be distressed and turn to drink, I focused on soothing her so that she did not cry.

Before he sobered up, he planned exciting day trip outings for when you were with us and he focused on you, Leo, but his sobriety coincided with the birth of Lilly and from then on, he focused totally on her. He was so delighted to have a baby daughter that it seemed to eclipse everything else. I am sure he was the same with you when you were a baby, but I was not there to witness that. What I am really trying to say is that although your dad sobering up was the best thing to happen, as he would have drunk himself to death, it changed the whole dynamics of the family. This coupled with the birth of Lilly seems to have meant that you and the other kids took a back seat. Indeed, one of the principles of AA is that the alcoholic has to be selfish. His sobriety must come first in every situation. To an extent this is true, as an alcoholic is only ever one drink away from drunk, but it requires patience to live with someone who has to be so selfish. Stopping drinking is not the end of the road; indeed, it is just the beginning and staying stopped is the goal.

There are some people who may disagree with me and you may be one of them, but I think that one of the main reasons that your dad turned to drink is that he is on the Autism Spectrum and he used alcohol to self-medicate and make himself feel normal. (It still does not make it right, of course.) He has never been officially diagnosed with Asperger's Syndrome or ASD (Autism Spectrum Disorder) or ADHD, but since your little brother Callum was diagnosed with ASD and we have learned more about the disorder, your dad sure seems to fit the bill! One of the giveaways is the hands over the ears when he hears any noise that bothers him and leaving the house when a baby cries. He certainly has some SPDs (Sensory Processing Disorders). There are certain noises that he cannot bear and he is super sensitive to touch. Leo, your dad has always been a keen timekeeper, but it is a little unusual to leave a doctor's appointment one minute after the specified appointment time has elapsed with the words, "Well, he is obviously not going to see me now, so I'm off."

I can't count the number of times your dad has told me that we are leaving for a family trip at a certain time and if we go past that time by even one second, he will calmly hang up the car keys and either turn on his computer or go to bed. I have learned to just carry on without him, as I have never been able to change his mind and persuade him to come. On other occasions, he has left without a member of the family, assuming that if they are not ready at the specified time that they do not wish to come along. However this is not a letter about your dad; it is about you and me. I guess I am just trying to explain to you what our everyday life has been like. It has had lots of highs and lows. There have been times when I have thought that we would not make it as a couple. The longer I am with your dad, the more I get to know him, but of course, one cannot ever truly know another person. In the earlier days of our marriage, I did not really know him at all because his true personality was masked by alcohol. Then in the early alcohol-free days, he found life very difficult as he began to face the reality of life. The turning point in his life, my life, and our marriage was when we became Christians in 2001. As I get to know him better, I find that he is an exceptionally generous and loyal man who loves God and his family more than anything else in the world.

Still you were not really part of our everyday life and in some ways you got the best deal as your visits always occurred during the school holidays. I was a teacher so could look after you then. We had some good holidays including going to Malta and several trips to the Lake District. A few times, we just went to my mum's house in Wales. Your dad organized a holiday for you and Lilly to Disneyland Paris again, but you arrived without your passport. I am pretty sure that it was deliberate as you did not want to go, but at the time I was really sorry for you as I thought it was an honest mistake. It turned out that the trip did not go ahead anyway as Lilly had severe toothache and Callum had chicken pox so we got our money back.

I hope that as you look back at your life, you will have some good memories of the early years of your dad's marriage to me before drugs and eventually heroin took a hold of your life.

In January 2001, an event occurred that was a defining moment in my life. I came to the point where I could no longer cope with Daniel's choices to abuse alcohol and drugs and his total disregard for discipline both at home and at school and I made the decision to turn him over to social services. This broke my heart.

You may remember that the Christmas before had been a total wash-out. There is a photo somewhere of the three of you (Daniel, Sally, and yourself) standing next to each other wearing WWF T-shirts and smiling to the camera. You all look happy, but this belies what was really going on, as you and Daniel were probably stoned and Sally was majorly traumatized, as at the end of the previous year I had sent her to live with my mum for seven weeks after she had a huge argument with your dad. During the time she was away, I had a miscarriage and when she returned, your dad had walked out on me for a week. We were now all back together, but on really shaky ground. We had just moved to a house near to Daniel and Sally's school, which your dad had chosen. The move was supposed to signal a new beginning for us all, not least for Daniel as he had started to get into a lot of trouble with the police. Your dad was now paying the mortgage and taking his financial responsibilities very seriously and you were down to stay with us for Christmas. Your dad had forbidden you to leave the house or go out with Daniel. Daniel was also supposed to stay in, but managed to get out once to meet one of his friends. We knew that he had started to smoke cannabis and he kept insisting that you did, too, and that you had introduced him to cannabis when he stayed with you and your mum some eighteen months previously. You, of course, denied it. Sally also kept telling me that you used drugs, but your behavior was different than Daniel's. You were not rude or aggressive and generally towed the line, at least when you were with us. It appears that Daniel and you were actually smoking dope upstairs in the bedroom you shared for much of that holiday. You had brought a lot with you and Daniel spent all the money he got for Christmas on drugs. How little I knew! I just knew that both of you seemed tired all the time and didn't really want to participate with the rest of the family.

The house was still not completely unpacked and there were boxes stacked in the conservatory. I had put up a Christmas tree, but was still suffering from post-natal depression, which had been made worse by events leading up to our move. So on the outside everything looked rosy, but things were about to explode.

After Daniel left, or more accurately after I kicked him out of the family home, I was really in a state of total depression and went on to have a breakdown that resulted in me getting early retirement from teaching. I truly wanted my life to end and felt like a complete failure as a mother. So really when I became a Christian, I realized that I could not make it on my own.

From this point on, your visits were very different. Daniel was sometimes with us and sometimes not. After we became Christians, he started to come back on overnight stays and eventually left his foster home to come back to live with us the following August. From then on, he was back and forth between living at our house and living at his friend's house. We only had one rule for him and that was no alcohol or drugs in your body or on your person. He would, of course, agree to the rule, come back, and then break it and the cycle would start again.

"What has this got to do with me?" you might ask, as you were not living with us and still only coming on visits. I guess the only thing it has to do with you is that because we never caught you with drugs, you were allowed to stay in our house whereas Daniel was not. Daniel and Sally always saw this as a travesty of justice. I tried to follow up their claims and your dad spoke to his parents and brother Andreas, but everything was hotly denied and you even wrote me a long letter assuring me that you were not taking any drugs and that you never had taken any and that all allegations were untrue. I know now that they were true, but at the time had to accept your version. This has been a hard thing for me to get over. In actual fact, I was glad that you were never caught with drugs, as I did not wish for your dad to ban you from our house—one alienated son was enough—nevertheless the lies cut me deeply.

Your visits became less and less frequent as you got older, but you always seemed to come at Christmas. For a couple of years, you came with a friend called Doug and again the visits were sad for me as Daniel would never come home for Christmas as he said he refused to play happy families just to make me feel better at Christmas. He often used to ask me if he could stay the night at other times, but, as I knew he was drinking and smoking cannabis, I had to say no, because your dad was very strict about the no-alcohol and no-drugs rule. You, however, were allowed to stay. The Bible is right when it says, "Love covers a multitude of sins." As natural parents, we are more prone to overlook and forgive our own children than we are to do the same for our stepchildren.

I think your visits became less frequent because as you got older, you were starting to live your own life, and maybe also because your dad had stopped drinking and in a way become less *fun* and a lot more serious. In 2003, Callum was born, so now you had two half-siblings to contend with and toddlers and teens don't mix very well. Only you can know why you came less often. Visits were planned and then at the last minute cancelled. I think that the last visit you had before we came to Australia, I was not even there. You came down with a girlfriend and I remember making up beds for you and her in separate bedrooms before I went to my mum's for the weekend. Your dad then rang me and said that because he had insisted that you could not sleep together, you had left and gone to stay in a hotel in Chester.

Our decision to come to Australia was very sudden. It is not a place either your dad or I had ever wanted to live. We had actually been in the process of applying for residency in Canada, as that was a place that we both loved, but Australia? It was not even on our radar. I think your dad asked you if you wanted to come, but I am not sure. You did not even want to come on visits anymore and I think I just figured that you would not even miss us. You seemed very settled. You had a job, a car, a girlfriend, and I seem to remember that you were even doing some studying. We thought you were happy and that you didn't want much to do with us when we left. I am sorry if you felt abandoned by us. In fact to this day, I still don't know how you felt because you rarely talk about your feelings.

Of course, after we got to Australia, we realized that things were not going so well with you as every time your dad tried to ring you, you were always "in bed sleeping" and refused to speak to him. Your dad was really hurt by this and was ready to give up on contacting you, but I encouraged him to always keep a door open to you. He wrote you a letter, but had no reply. I continued to get in touch from time to time and sent you birthday and Christmas presents and letters with no response. Then your dad had news from your mum that she was really worried because you were using heroin. Our son, a heroin addict—this was a big shock to us. Leo, I can tell you that you were never out of our prayers during those years. We lived in constant fear that we would receive a call on the phone to say that either you or Daniel was dead. I prayed for you every day and you were constantly in our thoughts. There did not seem to be any hope for your future.

So, Leo, you were absent, but not forgotten. Certainly we could have done things differently. Maybe things would have been better, only God knows, but be assured I made a choice to love you when I married your dad and I care what happens to you.

Laura

LETTER 2

You Tube

Dear Leo,

I am writing to you now because I am so proud of you and what you have become. None of the credit goes to me, of course, unless you count praying for you as deserving of credit. I have just watched the post on "You Tube" where you give a little of your life story. It is truly amazing how much you have changed.

I feel some guilt that I wasn't there for you enough when you were a teenager, so looking at the "You Tube" video and hearing you speak about those years made me want to cry. I am so happy that you have conquered your addiction to heroin and methadone. Your story is amazing. I am also glad that your dad and I were able to be with you through the first few weeks of your methadone withdrawal (after your initial cold turkey experience, which must have been hell on earth to go through). I remember the phone call that your dad had from Grandma saying that you had decided to quit methadone cold turkey, that it was dangerous, and that it was our fault. We had been so shocked when we arrived in the United Kingdom and saw you for the first time in four years. We had not realized that you were so reliant on methadone or really that it was a replacement addiction. We had been so happy to be in communication with you again and so over the moon that you had made a decision to become a Christian that we did not really realize or know what was really going on in your day-to-day life.

Getting back to the phone call, your dad came off the phone and basically said that if anything went wrong with the withdrawal, it would be my fault as I was the one who had prompted him to tell you that unless you came off methadone, we would not want you to come and visit us in Australia.

Leo, it was not only my decision; it was also your dad's. We realized that you would not be able to get a visa whilst on methadone and we also realized when we met you that it still wasn't the real you. Sometimes, I forget how direct and instant your dad is and had not realized that he had just bluntly told you that you needed to come off methadone before you could come and visit us.

To this day, I am not sure if this was what triggered you to attempt the cold turkey, but that is what it seemed like to us. Whatever the case, we certainly prayed for you and I can only imagine what dedication and love was shown to you by the people that helped you through those first ten days. It was truly amazing how it came to be that we were in the United Kingdom with you at that time. Now to see you on "You Tube" sharing a little of your life story and showing how much your life has changed is really encouraging.

Yesterday, we got the news that your visitor's visa to Australia has been granted and that you will now be able to come and visit us here in Australia. This is nothing short of a miracle with your drug-related police record. God is so good. I know that the prospect of you coming here has really made your father a very happy man. I know that he would like it to be more long term, but we will just have to see how things pan out.

I am a little nervous about the trip because it will take a bit of adjustment for us all to be living under the same roof. As you know, Sally is back living with us, and this has also been an adjustment for us all. It helps me to appreciate how your father must feel as Sally is not his natural daughter and so there is always that tension and feeling of divided loyalties. Often as a stepparent, you feel excluded from the natural parent-child relationship, but you have to step into the shoes of being a parent to a child that is not your own and of course, who has their own mother/father who you in no way replace. Relationships take time and commitment. So I am nervous, but also excited to have you back with us, this time in Australia.

Laura

LETTER 3

Part of the Family

Wow, Leo,

The time has come for us to say goodbye to you once again. These last seven months have been a truly memorable time for us. Although I was very happy at the prospect of you coming here to stay with us, I must admit that I was also quite anxious about how it would all work out. We have never been together for that amount of time before and I knew that your dad would be working for the majority of the time you spent in Australia. (Hmm . . . some things never change!) I knew that I personally would be spending a lot of time with you when your dad was at work, Lilly and Callum were at school, and Sally was at work. This made me a little nervous as I often have a very long day, getting up at 5:00 a.m. to spend some time with your dad before he goes to work and often not in my own bed before 12:00 a.m. as I settle Callum and Lilly for the night and clear up the house ready for another day. So the time that the children are at school is very precious to me, as the rest of the time I am *giving out* and that is the time that I recharge my batteries. With you in the house, I knew I was not going to be able to fully relax. For the past year and a half, we have been dealing with a difficult situation here at home with Sally coming back to live with us. As you know, she has suffered trauma and is still recovering.

To be truthful, I did not really know what it would be like with you living with us. My only real experience of any extended time with you was when we spent time with you on our first trip back to the United Kingdom when your grandpa first became so ill and this included the month in Ireland following your cold turkey from methadone. The stay in Ireland was a really hard time for everyone. Physically and emotionally, you were a wreck, and again, I was in charge with your dad working. Callum and Lilly were missing school so I was trying to homeschool them in the mornings. It poured with rain every single day, the weather was becoming colder, there was no Internet connection in the chalet, and I couldn't get any credit on my phone, so I personally felt cut off from the world. Your dad left really early for work and I had to drive him there. Callum would not stay in the chalet with you and Lilly so I had to wake him early every morning to get in the car with your dad and me. This, of course, meant that I had no respite from him. To top it all off, Callum and I got the flu so I ended up having him with me in bed and your dad had his room. All in all, I could not wait to leave Ireland. It is only in retrospect that I can see God's hand in our stay there as we were so cut off from everyone and everything we knew that it meant that you were not confronted by old friends who were still using heroin or were on methadone. You were completely away from your old stomping grounds and spent a lot of the time just sitting reading your Bible. We got a little bit of sightseeing in and I reckon we saw everything there was to see in Cork, even if it was through sheets of rain! Nevertheless, I found those weeks really difficult. You had a lot of bad body odor as you were obviously still sweating out some of the bad effects of the methadone. You were also constantly shaking, which meant that the car was shaking when you were in it and also the dining table used to wobble as you were constantly shaking your legs underneath it. Of course, I have no idea what it must have been like for you having gone through the intense withdrawal symptoms up in Scotland to then find yourself in Ireland with your dad, your stepmother, your half-sister, and your half-brother, not forgetting that your stepbrother is autistic and that is a whole other ball game. I am sure that I am not an easy person to live with sometimes.

I did not get any respite because, of course, as soon as your dad came back from work, you both wanted to spend time with each other and used to go and sit in the foyer of the main hotel. So the point of me remembering this is that it made me apprehensive about your stay in Australia.

I guess what I am trying to say is that I did not really know you as a person so didn't know what it would be like having you to live with us. The girls were quite anxious about having a strange man in the house even if that man was their brother. Callum did not say how he was feeling, but then, being autistic, he struggles with his emotions and so I just prepared him with the facts of you coming, which he accepted. Callum and Lilly had time to get to know the new you a little better because we had just returned to the United Kingdom and spent nearly two months with you there and in Italy. Sally was another matter and she was the most apprehensive; all she remembered was you as a teenager.

Now that the visit has happened and the seven months are over, I am overwhelmed with emotion. As I said, when I married your dad, I chose to love you as his son; now I love you for who you are. God has been really gracious to me and given me a love for you that transcends that of stepparent, or at least of how I chose to love you before. I am truly sad to see you go and will have many great memories of your time with us. At first, I found it a bit awkward having you in the house. I had to get used to wearing my dressing gown all the time or getting dressed before leaving my bedroom. I had to get used to never being alone in the house and to feeling that another adult was watching every moment of my parenting and seeing firsthand the relationship I have with your dad. That is how it felt at first and I found it quite hard.

However, over the months I have managed to relax a little and have been able to see some of your very admirable qualities. Leo, one of the best things about you is your ability to mind your own business. I am sure there have been many occasions you wanted to comment on the way I do things or the way your dad does things, but you just mind your own business. You don't tell me how to bring up Lilly and Callum and point out ways I could do it better. You don't tell me how to run my house, or point out ways I could do it better. If you disapprove of what I do or how I do it, you don't say. This is an amazing quality, Leo, and is one you should foster and develop.

I have also been amazed at your willingness to help around the house and around the garden. Thank you so much for all your gardening; it has been so much appreciated. It has been really good spending time with you on your own and also with the family. Sally and Lilly both love you to death. You have completely won them over. They will miss you so much over the coming months and possibly years, as who knows what the future holds? Callum has not been able to say it, but he will miss you, too. You have been amazing with him: patient and kind. Our trampoline has never seen so much use. Callum has always loved it, but with you available to join in, or to watch him, it has been so much more fun. I am sure there were many times when jumping on the trampoline with your little brother would not have been your first choice of activity, but you still joined in. Not forgetting that when we had to move halfway through your stay, you dismantled and reassembled the trampoline. This was a feat that had been beyond two removal men, but you managed it single-handedly!

Thank you also for the many times you have looked after him, enabling your dad and me to have some time together. We never usually get time alone and it has been wonderful.

I have seen your dad come to life with you over here. This in itself is reward enough. He has been surprised at how much he has enjoyed you being here and also at how much he has already started to miss you. He told me the other day that as he was coming home from work, he got a sinking feeling in the pit of his stomach as he realized that you were not going to be there. He even said that he got a taste of what it must be like for your grandma now that your grandpa has died, returning to the house and not finding him there. This brings me of course, to the death of your grandpa. As you know, we returned again to the United Kingdom for your grandparent's fiftieth wedding anniversary celebration and also for the wedding of my cousin Carol's son. It was an amazing visit and we even got to spend a week in Italy with you and Daniel. So once again, we spent time in Scotland with your family and in Wales with my mum. My sister even had the chance to come over for a couple of weeks. (The whole of last year was full of family reunions; we have been so blessed.) We realized when we were in Scotland that your grandpa was not going to be around for much longer as he seemed to get weaker each day we were there. It is, of course, a miracle that he survived his liver cancer for so long, having been given only two weeks to live the first time we came back. To have lasted another two years is amazing. We wondered if he would pass away before we returned to Australia with you, but he did not. I imagine it must have been sad for you to leave him, knowing how ill he was and facing the possibility that you would never see him again in this life. I know that the last goodbye was hard for your dad.

Modern technology is amazing, isn't it? With the use of Skype, you and your dad were able to be with your grandpa for the last week of his life, even though he was in Scotland and you were in Australia. It shows another depth to your character that you were able to keep a vigil for your grandpa for the last week of his life. You even slept on the couch in front of the computer so that you could be *near* him. It was an emotionally charged week and you remained faithful and encouraging to both your grandpa and grandma throughout, as well as to other members of your family as they visited with your grandpa. So that is another memory that I have of your visit here. It was sad that your grandpa's life ended, but we believe that he is now in heaven and the sadness is only for those who remain, especially your grandma who will miss him every second of the day. I could not stay in front of the Skype camera for long, as seeing your grandpa dying reminded me of the death of my own father, but I was glad to be able to say my goodbyes and I was glad that your dad could *be with* his own dad and mum during that time. I know that your dad got to say a lot of things to his own father, as he lay on his deathbed, that he needed to say, and that was a good thing. I know when my dad died, I felt we had a lot of unfinished business, but I think that your own dad is at peace with the death of your grandpa.

At church last Sunday, someone asked me how everything was since you had gone. I felt tears well up in my eyes, so the answer is we miss you. For me, this is truly amazing because I never would have dreamed that I would feel this way. It is more than just missing you; it is the fact that it signals the end of our family reunion. Goodness only knows how I will feel when Daniel has to return. Lilly said I should not feel sad, just happy that you were able to come, and that we were able to be together as a family. Most of the time, I can do that.

So—it's all about the *memories.* Here are some of mine of you: The zany sayings, fizzing, and clicking; the midnight smoothie making; the day in the city followed by the Dorian buying; talk about the power of suggestion; the honey (definitely the honey, especially you packing the bee-power honey and bee pollen mixture in your suitcase to take back); the pancakes, baked beans and warm mangoes (not as a combo); the bike riding, sunbathing, swimming and gym workouts; your birthday barbeque; days at the beach (especially the Palm Beach saga of the lost keys); training the puppy; the chai lattes and Boost Juices; family board game night; the Christmas you didn't want to celebrate, but did for us (thank you); the banter between you and Daniel: the quiet Bible reading and late night DVD watching; the wedding vows renewal day at the beach and testimony nights at the church; the packing and unpacking; and last but not least the Leo trail that you left around the house of T-shirts, towels, shoes, backpacks, books, laptops, phones, hats, and socks.

I look forward to seeing you grow and mature as both a person and a Christian and I wish for you a good wife. As you said in your prayer on the day you left, we thank God that he has restored the years that the locusts have eaten and that our family is reconciled.

Love,

Laura

P.S. How could I forget to mention one of the things I will remember most is the sight of you and your dad in your kilts?

4

To the Children of My Second Marriage

A Baby at Forty!

Dear Lilly,

Well, I never thought in a million years that I would again be giving birth! Your birth must go down as one of the most celebratory moments of my life. Of course, the birth of any child is extraordinary and a cause for joy and celebration, but for me personally, your birth had a special significance. When I fell pregnant with you only a few months after I married your dad, it was such a surprise! Your dad and I met in London, which is strange as neither of us are Londoners. Let me tell you about that before I get on to your actual birth because it will give you a little background into our relationship and also help you to see why your birth was so amazing!

As you know, your dad is not the father of Daniel and Sally. Their father was my first husband. We were divorced and we had been separated for over six years when I met your dad.

After living and working in Stoke-on-Trent for ten years, I had ended up back in London after my dad died. My intention was to help Daniel and Sally build a relationship with their real father. I wanted them to have family around them and to be part of their father's extended family even if we were not still together. It seemed that my family was dwindling, with my dad dead and my sister, as ever, so far away. Lone parenting had been hard and very lonely and my dad's death had really made me think about the importance of relationships, my own mortality, and the brevity of life. I wanted your older brother and sister to have a chance at happiness and good relationships. I had come to realize that in the end, family is all there is. It is the unit that holds society and indeed countries together.

The move to London was an adventure and in some ways quite reckless. I had applied for two teaching jobs in South East London and was offered one of them. The position was at an all boys secondary school. After accepting the job as Head of Department, I leased out my house in Stoke and rented a house in South East London. As is usual with me, it all happened quite quickly. My dad died in November 1995 and by the following July, I was upping sticks and relocating back to South East London, near to Daniel and Sally's father's family. I was also back to where I had spent many years at Teacher Training College and where I had lived whilst working briefly in central London as an audio secretary and for many years at my first teaching job in a boy's school in Brixton. I had, in fact, heard about the job through an old friend from my teaching days in Brixton who was now working at the school where I got the job.

Lilly, after my first marriage broke up the last thing on my mind was re-marriage or even dating. I was truly disillusioned about my chances at a successful romantic relationship and I felt the time had come for me to progress in my career and look after my children. For them, it was probably the most stable period of their lives and for that, at least, I am grateful. After my dad died, I went a bit crazy and I briefly dated a few guys I met mainly at nightclubs. Sadly, they were on the whole not really after meaningful relationships, just physical ones. When I moved to London, I decided that the time had come for me to start dating again, but where was I to meet men that were not just after a short-term physical relationship, but would be interested in me as a person?

There were lots of men at work, but they were all married, had girlfriends, or were gay. As I wasn't really after having an affair, I decided to join a dating agency. Yes, I know this may be a bit of a shock to you and perhaps the others as it is something your dad and I have kept relatively quiet. We met through a British Dating Agency called *Dateline*. It was not an online dating agency then. I do not know if it is now. It cost me two hundred pounds for my first year's membership and I had to fill in a long questionnaire about the type of person I was looking for and also about the type of person I was myself. Although I had to describe my looks, there were no photos to be sent. I told a few friends that I had joined (for safety reasons), but mostly I kept it to myself.

Your dad was the tenth man I met. What can I say? It was love at first sight. He was so cute and so attentive. He had short jelled hair and the most sparkling eyes I had ever seen and that voice, with that Scottish lilt—so gorgeous—I was completely captivated. The most fantastic thing about him was that he drank *water not alcohol.* So like I have always told you, we met at a train station. On that first date, we had KFC and went to a few pubs in South East London. All the while your dad drank water. The most amazing thing for me was that he wanted to see me again and soon. Most of the other guys I had met through dateline wanted to see me again and some were really nice men, but I was not attracted to any of them, so to be attracted to someone and have the feeling be mutual was wonderful.

Looking back, we should not really have been matched by the computer. I had stated I wanted someone who either did not drink or who only drank infrequently, on a social basis. I was not looking to have more children and I wanted someone to date not necessarily have a serious long- term relationship. Your dad on the other hand had asked for someone who liked to drink, who was looking for a long-term permanent relationship and who wanted more children, as he was really keen on having more children. So what happened there I do not know. It must have been because we both said we liked travelling and playing chess and the funny thing is that the last chess game we played was over thirteen years ago, before you were even born!

It was a whirlwind romance. Your dad pursued me with flowers, chocolates, gifts, letters, and phone calls. Within a few months, we moved in together and within five months we were married. We married in November 1997 and by the end of the year, I realized that my water-drinking husband was in fact another alcoholic in disguise. I loved him to bits and he was not at all like Daniel and Sally's father who drank every day. He was a binge drinker, which meant he could go for days, weeks, or even months without touching a drop and then he would go on an absolute bender, drinking twenty-four/seven for days, weeks or even months. I was far too embarrassed to tell any of my friends or family that there was a problem, I felt so stupid. I just pretended that there was no problem. Daniel and Sally were not, at first, aware, I don't think, as most of the drinking would be done when they were at their own dad's or with their grandparents. Also when your dad was drinking, he was a very benevolent drunk. He would basically take them down to the shops and treat them to whatever they wanted. He was usually generous and jovial, at least at the start of a binge. If the binge went on too long, he would retreat into himself and hide himself away and drink. He rarely appeared drunk and was usually very quiet.

When we got married, I had just bought a flat in South East London; your dad had just bought a flat in Surrey and I still owned the ex-council house in Stoke. We were living in the flat in South East London; the flat in Surrey was empty and the tenants in Stoke were not paying their rent. It was not an ideal situation and although your dad was solvent, I was getting deeper and deeper into debt. We decided to put all properties on the market and sell the first two that got buyers and live in the third. The flat in Surrey sold immediately; the flat in South East London took a few weeks and the house in Stoke remained unsold—so time to move back up north.

Believe it or not, Lilly, when I met your dad I was earning more than him. This being the case, I was still getting deeper and deeper into debt every month. I was paying two mortgages and not getting any rent returns from the house in Stoke. I was paying huge childcare fees for before- and after-school care for Daniel and Sally. Their dad had never really supported them financially, but did pay childcare fees for the first year after I moved back to London. From the day he found out that I was dating your father, he has never paid another penny in maintenance. When your dad and I first got married, our finances were in a bit of a mess. We never sat down and worked out who would pay for what. Your dad had been lodging with a family and just paying board and lodging so had no idea about the cost of living. He had a son (your brother, Leo) from his first marriage and paid maintenance, but most of his income was disposable and by that I mean that he was used to having huge amounts of spare cash to spend on whatever he liked: holidays, booze, etc. I, on the other hand, was well aware of the cost of living having struggled as a single parent for many years to work and raise two children on my own. So in the beginning, I tried to match your dad's spending. We did not have joint accounts and we tended to put in half each for stuff like furniture.

He, on the other hand, did not pay anything toward the two mortgages that I had, along with a car loan. I have never liked talking about money and was scared of joint accounts because my first husband had drunk most of my earnings along with his own. I was fiercely independent having been on my own for so long. In fact, money was not that much of an issue, except that your dad had more to spend on Leo than I had to spend on Daniel and Sally or even myself and we were not sharing the financial load evenly. Over the years, everything has more than evened out and as you know, your dad is a most generous man. As I sit and write this letter now, thirteen years on, I am no longer teaching, his earnings have taken off, and he supports the family entirely, however at the time, it was an issue. I was keen to continue to progress in my career and was beginning to gain confidence in my abilities as a teacher. The school I was working at had an OFSTED inspection and my department came out very well in the inspection. Our school was linked to a nearby university for training student teachers; they were also due to undergo an OFSTED inspection. As part of that, I was individually assessed, as I trained a student teacher at the school. It was a huge responsibility and a lot of pressure. So as you can see, it probably was not the *right* time for me to get pregnant. I was newly married, at a crucial time in my career, and nearly forty with two children of my own already and one stepson. To top it all, hubby number two was another alcoholic.

All I can say is: God knew differently. His timing is perfect and that makes the timing of your birth perfect!

Back to the story, before I knew I was pregnant we sold the two flats in London, and so that meant we both had to look for work up north. I applied for a job in Cheshire, got an interview, and got the job. It all just seemed to fall into place. The school was due to have an OFSTED inspection, the department I was to head was in a mess, and they wanted me to come along and fix it. I was very pleased that everything seemed to be working out so well, although I was a little nervous about moving back up north because it would mean that Daniel and Sally would no longer be seeing their dad every other weekend. Your dad got a job in Northampton, which meant that he would have to live away during the week, but at least he would be nearer than London. At the time, I was taking the contraceptive pill.

One morning, I reached into the cupboard in the bathroom, which was strategically placed above the toilet, and accidentally dropped my packet of contraceptive pills into the toilet. I fished them out and threw them away and made an appointment to go and see the doctor for a new prescription. Within a couple of days, I had a new prescription and I waited for my period to come so that I could start taking the new pack.

That period never came; instead, my darling, you arrived nine months later.

When I told your dad I was pregnant, he was overjoyed. He had always wanted more children so was absolutely over the moon that it had happened so quickly. My emotions, on the other hand, were very mixed. Excitement and joy were mixed with a certain sense of trepidation, new stressful job, new (drinking) husband, big house move, and no support from family forthcoming, as your dad's family all live in Scotland and my mum was still very much grieving my dad's death. It was all rather scary and I was worried about Daniel and Sally and how the changes would affect them. They, particularly Daniel, had not adapted, at first, to the move down to London and it seemed that they had only just really begun to settle in. Daniel had started high school and so would have to move school and I was going to do all this whilst pregnant and then with a baby. My new husband would be working away from home all week—hmm, looked a bit like I was going to be a single parent again. Your dad was as ever optimistic. We would employ a nanny, I would be able to continue working, and the nanny would take the load off me. Simple!

Then all the bad news regarding the pregnancy began. I had a phone call from the hospital to come in and see them urgently. Blood tests had indicated that there was a high chance that my baby—you—would be Down syndrome. Along the way, further tests and scans were all pointing in that direction. The medical staff was convinced that I was having a Down's syndrome baby. Your father, conversely, was convinced that I was not. The pregnancy was not a smooth one. I had a blood test that went wrong and ended up with my arm in a sling for a couple of months just at the time when we were moving. I started my new job six months pregnant and, I must say, my new employers were not overjoyed at the situation, as it looked like my maternity leave could coincide with the up and coming OFSTED inspection.

Some amazing things happened whilst I was pregnant with you, Lilly. The most amazing thing that happened is that two months before you were born, your dad gave up drinking and he has not had a drop of alcohol ever since. He was determined that his new baby would never see him drunk. That is how much he was looking forward to your birth and how much he has loved you since before you were born.

Your dad's last year of drinking, which coincided with our first year of marriage, is a story in itself, full of trauma, tragedy, trials, and tears, but finally triumph. It does not really belong here in this letter because with you came a new beginning. Your older brothers and sister were part of that story.

Your dad, being the Scotsman that he is, was determined that you would be born in Scotland. He did not want you to be born in England. So I dutifully went along with his desires. I had all my maternity care in England, first in London, then in Stoke, but I booked into the Borders General Hospital for your birth. You were due on Christmas day! It was not possible for our whole family to stay at your grandma's whilst I waited for you to be born, so I arranged for Sally to spend a couple of weeks with Nana in Wales over Christmas and Daniel went down to London to be with his dad and his dad's family. For the second time in my life, I celebrated an early Christmas. Before your dad and I went up to Scotland and Daniel and Sally went off, we had Christmas dinner with all the trimmings and presents two weeks early. It reminded me of the early celebrations we had the year my dad died, but this time it was not a sad occasion, but more of a happy one. Recently, I saw a photograph of that day come up on the digital photo display that dad has running on his computer as a screen saver. Sally was eleven and Daniel was twelve. We were sitting at the table in the dining section of the living room of the house in Stoke. I was very skinny, but heavily pregnant and sporting a ring that your dad had bought me on a whirlwind shopping trip to the shopping center at Birmingham station. He had given me about sixty seconds to choose the ring. This is an impossible thing for me to do, so I just picked one that was on a special offer—a bargain. Sally and Daniel look happy, but I don't know now if they were.

I was very happy on that day. Your dad had stopped drinking after a near-death experience and he was off work recovering, so we were able to spend a lot of time together. Daniel and Sally had settled back into school. Sally had returned to her old primary school and I had managed to get Daniel into the best secondary school in the area, which was also one of the top comprehensive schools in the country. A few of his old friends were there and I believed he would do very well there.

Your dad and I travelled up to Scotland about a week before Christmas, after we had taken Sally to Wales and sent Daniel to London on the train to be met by his dad at the other end. On the outside, I was calm and seemingly okay, but inside I was really starting to panic. On previous occasions when we had been to Scotland, your dad had always ended up going on a complete drinking bender. On one occasion earlier that year, we had flown up to Scotland and he was so drunk by the time the plane got to Edinburgh airport that he ran away from me and I ended up getting straight back on a plane to London. It was supposed to have been a romantic weekend away for the two of us as Daniel and Sally were at their dad's, but instead it turned into a nightmare as we missed our flight. (Can you believe your dad was actually late? And that it was his fault, not mine?) We had to spend the night at the airport waiting for the next available flight. Of course, your dad had already started to celebrate his weekend away before we even got on the train to get to the airport, so now he was on a mission to consume as much alcohol as was humanly possible to imbibe before catching the next flight. I, on the other hand, was pregnant, exhausted from a week's teaching, and hungry. However, now that your dad was with his best friend and lover—alcohol—my needs were no longer his concern.

Looking back, I should have returned home at that point, but I thought things would get better once we arrived in Scotland. I do not know to this day what your dad got up to that weekend, apart from drinking nonstop, as we did not communicate whilst he was there and when he returned to London a few days later, he was still on his bender, even at this point starting to take bottles of vodka in his bag to work. I do know that it was one of the benders that actually made him realize that he needed to do something about his drinking before he killed himself, so in that sense it was a good thing. At Al Anon, I remember learning that crises are in fact good; they should be welcomed not avoided as they provide occasions for changed behavior and attitudes, both in the alcoholic and more importantly for me, in the person living with the alcoholic. Still because of this and other occasions, I was filled with dread returning to Scotland, especially as it was the festive season. What better excuse for a drink than Christmas, the birth of a new baby, and New Year in Scotland?

I was in fact absolutely petrified that once I had given birth your dad would not be able to resist celebrating/drowning his sorrows with all his old mates and that that would be the end of that, our marriage and everything else. His recovery would be well and truly over; he would be on one final never-ending bender. There would be wine, women, and song for him, probably ending in his death and I would be alone again, a single parent, but this time with a Down's syndrome baby and two older children on the cusp of becoming teenagers. I had constant nightmares that this would happen and I used to wake up in sweats of sheer terror. But like I said, on the outside I was calm, peaceful, and contented. (Sometimes, I think that I should have been an actor not a teacher, because I became adept at hiding the way I truly felt.) I know now that it was my past experiences that made me feel that way.

> As a pregnant eighteen year old, I felt abandoned by my own parents.
>
> I had been left in hospital alone for many days when Daniel was born whilst his dad went out drinking with his mates.
>
> When Sally was born, her dad moved out so that he could drink and pursue a sexual relationship with a female student.

So even though I had felt so happy at the Christmas celebrations with Daniel and Sally, the dread was well and truly taking hold. You were actually due on Christmas day, but like the others (and most babies) you decided not to come on the day you were expected. On the twenty-seventh, I went to the BGH hospital for a final scan and to be booked in for the next day. It was then I learned that you were going to be a girl. Your dad was so delighted, and he just could not believe it. He was absolutely over the moon. He had been convinced that you would be a boy and that he would never have a daughter of his own. Having five brothers and a son already, he really wanted a girl. We were going to call you Leroy after your dad, but as you were a girl, we had to change it to Lilly, which is nearly the same. (Okay, it starts and ends with the same letters!) I would have been happy for a boy or a girl as I already had one of each. I just wanted a healthy baby, and a present and sober dad.

The day of your arrival came; your dad and I went to the hospital and I was duly booked in. I was given drugs to induce labor, and from then on in your dad and I just hung about the hospital, taking walks and talking. In the afternoon, I decided to have a bath to see if that would get things started, but it wasn't until the early evening that I started to feel any labor pains. My cervix was slow to dilate, but by about 8:00 p.m., I was in labor. Three hours and fifteen minutes later, you were born. The actual birth was very fast and your poor dad nearly had to deliver you by himself as the midwife left the room briefly, but she soon returned when she heard your dad's cries of help. I couldn't wait to see you. I already knew that you were a girl, but were you Down's syndrome? The moment I saw you, I fell in love again. You were not Down's syndrome, but you know even if you had been, I would still have loved you just as much; it is a magical thing, motherhood and birth. You love the child no matter what. However, as it happens, I was expecting you to be Down's syndrome, but you were not, and your birth rates as one of the most exhilarating moments in my life. You were a little smaller than the first two, but still average. Your hair was dark and that was a surprise to me as my other two had been blond babies, almost hairless in fact. I don't think Sally had proper hair until she was three or four years old; it was just like a wispy, fine down on her head. Yours was definitely hair. You were born at 11:15 p.m. and shortly afterwards, your dad went to Grandma's to get some sleep. He had stayed with me all through the labor. He did not abandon me and start to drink. Early next morning, he was back and very loving and attentive to both you and I. It was amazing; my fears began to subside as your dad proved that he was sober and was going to stay sober.

I stayed in hospital for a few days just so that the two of us could get used to each other and I could recover a little from the birth. Your dad was with me all the time, only leaving to get a few hours of kip. All the staff at the hospital thought that it was very patriotic of your dad to want you to be born in Scotland so that you could be his "wee Scottish bairn."

On the thirty-first of December 1998, I was discharged from the hospital, with you in my arms and dad by my side. Instead of your dad going to the pub to celebrate (wet the baby's head) we all went to Grandma's and some of his family and a couple of his friends came over to welcome you into the world. It was all very sedate and there was no alcohol to be seen. You were admired by all and cuddled by a few honored people. (Even then your dad was very protective over you.) Daniel and Sally were due back on January 2 and we decided to travel back to Stoke–on–Trent that evening (New Years Eve 1998).

I knew that on previous years, this would have been a huge drinking event for your dad because as you know New Year is a bigger celebration in Scotland than Christmas, but he wasn't even remotely interested in that, only in you, his darling wee daughter. It was a new experience for me, too, to have a husband that was so attentive to the new baby and also to me.

We ended up leaving very late in the evening, about 11:30 p.m., if my memory serves me correctly. The journey down to Stoke was stressful as you were a new baby and needed feeding a couple of times en route. Unbeknown to us all, the service stations on the motorways were closed from 12:00 p.m. to 6:00 a.m. New Year's Day. We had not accounted for this—but we survived!

My fears surrounding your birth were unfounded. Your dad did not go on a bender. I was not left all alone in the hospital. Your dad did not leave me. You were not Down's syndrome. I survived giving birth at age forty-and-a-half. Things were indeed looking up! Best of all, your dad was so excited and delighted that you were a girl. He had been right all along—there was nothing wrong with you at all.

Love,

Mum

xxxx

P.S. Hope this gives you some idea of how much you mean to your dad and me. We still feel exactly the same about you now.

LETTER 2

Allergies Emerge

Dear Lilly,

You of all people are aware of your allergies now, but it was a slow learning curve for your dad and me. We had a few scares along the way, but like everything else, it teaches you something. Each scare reminds us how precious you are to us, and how we do not want anything bad to happen to you.

The first indication we had that you were going to suffer from allergies was your skin. From birth you had very dry skin, which at first we thought was because you were an overdue baby, as I had heard that this could cause the newborn to have dry skin. I soon realized that it was more than this as your skin easily became red and inflamed and often looked very sore. You were quickly diagnosed as having atopic eczema. Your dad, being a keen researcher, quickly discovered all the things we could do to make you more comfortable. Firstly, we got rid of all of your clothes that were not pure cotton. I changed my washing detergent to one for sensitive skin. I stopped wearing perfume or spray on deodorant and we gave our cat away. (Giving the cat away made me very sad, but it was worth it because it would have made you even more uncomfortable if we had kept him.) His name was Ginger and he was really Daniel's cat.

The second indication we had that your allergies were not isolated to skin irritation is when I started to wean you. I was planning on going back to work, so when you were about four months old, I started to give you formula milk as well as breast milk. It was then that the projectile vomiting and diarrhea started. It really took me by surprise and at first I thought you had some sort of virus, but soon realized it was related to the formula milk. I took you to the doctor who prescribed you with Infasoy, which was a brand of formula soya milk. This did the trick and the vomiting stopped. I was told that you were intolerant to milk.

The third indication we had that feeding you was going to be a tricky business was when I decided to give you some lightly scrambled eggs. By this time, you were sitting in a high chair and I was putting the food on the tray in front of you. You being a pretty normal baby put your hands straight into the food during a moment's inattention on my part. The reaction was instant red welts started appearing on your hands and soon they were also on your face as you put your hands to your face. Everywhere that you touched went red. I immediately removed the eggs and then removed you from the chair, quickly immersing your hands and arms under water and washed your face. You did not seem to be upset at all, but it scared me so it was off to the doctor's again. This time he decided to do a blood test and check for allergies. The results showed that you did indeed have an allergy to eggs. Of course, I now know that you also have many other allergies and I have often wondered why at that time, this was not more fully investigated. Knowing a bit more about allergies now, I would have assumed that this would be the natural thing to do. However, it wasn't and so we have almost had to discover each of your allergies only after you have suffered a reaction! At this point, your dad decided never to give you anything containing nuts, because although we had not been told that you had a nut allergy, he almost had a sixth sense that you were allergic to nuts because of your other allergies. I had avoided giving all my other children nuts before they were five, due to the fear of them choking, but this was different.

You continued to have quite severe reactions to foods and it was just really a matter of trial and error. The reactions were limited to redness and swelling of your skin and often resulted in hives and looked like severe nettle rash. I did keep taking you to the doctor and at one point; he said that you had a pattern of random reactions so I should just keep a close watch on you for symptoms. By this time, you were attending nursery as I was back at work, and they were avoiding giving you foods that contained eggs or milk. I would often get a call from nursery staff that would let me know that they had had to give you a cool bath as you had had a so-called "random reaction." (This was not cruel because it was also what I did at home and what I had asked them to do. It seemed to sooth you and resulted in the rashes subsiding.) Your eczema was also quite severe at this point, and I found it very difficult to keep your skin comfortable. You had difficulty sleeping and I spent most nights stripping you down to your nappy and applying soothing creams to your whole body over and over again. This, plus the massaging, would eventually get you to sleep. When you moved into your own little room, this meant that I had to put a quilt on the floor and lie with you there, as there was only a cot and a cupboard in the room. I often also played music softly in the background, as this also seemed to sooth you.

Your dad took immense pleasure from having you around and he did feed you and change your nappy sometimes. He also bathed you quite often, but I always had to be there as well. He loved to take you with him wherever he went when he was not at work, but when you were very little, he always insisted on me being there as well. In the early days, we often went for walks with you in the pram or I would strap you to me in a front sling. He also bought a baby-carrying seat that he could strap to his back and he loved to carry you in that. You also loved it and would stay in it happily whilst we were out and about.

Your dad doted on you, but was never one for getting up much in the night, so that all rested on me and as he could not cope with you crying, I could never *leave you to cry.* Most of the time, it would not have been appropriate to do this because you were crying due to discomfort from your eczema. I have to admit that this was very exhausting for me and I was always on edge and more or less jumped to your every need. On some occasions, when I could not soothe you quickly enough, your dad would run out of the house with his hands over his ears and drive off. This used to scare me and I could not understand it. Now I have come to realize that he has a Sensory Processing Disorder (SPD) and that he hears very differently from other people. Whereas most people find the sound of babies crying distressing, they are able to filter it out some-what, especially if they know that the baby is being attended to. For your dad, this is not the case; the sound simply overwhelms his whole being and he has to leave. This is the main reason that although he was happy to care for you and be with you, he always wanted me there in case you cried and he could not cope. I found this very difficult to understand or cope with. It meant that I could never fully relax and I am sure that it contributed to my depression. Due to your allergies, I was always on full alert anyway, but not being allowed to let you cry was very stressful as, my dear, all babies cry and you were no exception.

Fortunately, you were quite a good-natured little soul and were often very content. You had the most gorgeous blue eyes and beautiful smile and often strangers in the street would comment on your eyes. Every-one who met you liked you. As a baby and toddler, we took you to two AA retreats and you were the star of the show. Children were not usu-ally allowed, but they made an exception for you as you were so well behaved and just sat on my lap or on a blanket on the floor during all the sessions.

As you grew a little older, I used to let you have your bottle of soya milk in bed, contrary to all child-rearing advice, because quite simply it stopped you scratching and helped you to get to sleep and therefore I also got some sleep. I also let you have it in the car, in the pushchair; in fact, I always made sure that I had a couple of bottles of soya milk on hand.

I would say that your early years, although marred somewhat by having eczema and some food allergies, were very good. You were wanted and loved by both your parents. You did not lack for any material thing. If anything, your dad spoiled you with toys and gifts. It was sometimes hard for me because I saw the difference between the way your dad cared for you and the way that Sally and Daniel's dad cared for them. The difference was overwhelming and I knew that I could not make it up to them.

It was apparent from an early age that you were very bright. You loved books and any sort of craft. You particularly loved coloring tiny mosaic patterns and you and your dad would sit for hours and hours, coloring in opposite sides of mosaic pictures. You also loved to play on the piano and when my sister came from overseas to visit, would happily sit on her lap whilst she played.

Fortunately, you did not have an anaphylactic reaction until you were five. That sure was a shock when it happened! It was on your second visit to Canada. Callum was a baby and we had gone to visit an old school friend of mine in Ottawa. Sally had remained with your uncle and aunt and cousins in Peterborough and neither Leo nor Daniel had come with us on this trip. As luck would have it, on this occasion, I had persuaded your dad to take you on a trip by himself. You were no longer a baby and had started school so he felt a lot more confident that he could cope. He had also started taking you for swimming lessons on a Saturday morning in the United Kingdom, so was happy for it to be just the two of you, although he would have preferred for Callum and me to go as well.

He had wanted to go and visit Montreal and I thought the train trip would be too much for me to cope with because Callum was still a baby. I had already been to Montreal when I was in my early twenties and was happy to stay at my friend's house for the day with Callum. I needed a rest as we had been doing a lot of sightseeing in Ottawa and I was finding it exhausting with the baby and you.

To cut a long story short, not long after you got to Montreal, he took you to a food court for something to eat. He does not know what you ate or touched, but you had an anaphylactic reaction and he panicked. Fortunately, there was an English lady sitting opposite him whose two daughters had peanut allergies. Apparently she took over and got you some medical assistance. This was a miracle. It shows to me, God was looking after you even then. When you arrived back in Ottawa that evening your face was still very swollen and your dad was very shaken by the experience. I don't think that you saw much of Montreal! We assumed that you had touched or eaten something that contained nuts, as you had never had such a severe reaction from eggs. We determined to have you tested again for allergies on our return to the United Kingdom. This we did and discovered that you were strongly allergic to hazelnuts and walnuts and also allergic to other tree nuts. It was then that I realized the reason for the many reactions that you had started to have to chocolate. Although I had never given you chocolate containing nuts, you must have had some chocolate that stated on the label "may contain traces of nuts." It was at this stage that you were proscribed with antihistamines and an EpiPen and we were advised that you needed this emergency medication with you at all times.

What a trial that must seem to you sometimes, every journey or outing, however small, even walking the dog, or riding your scooter to the park and you have to carry your medicine bag. Of course, there have also been the panics when we have gone out and left your medicine at home or we have gone shopping and left it in a shop. Looking back, it is funny to think of the amount of times we have had to retrace our steps to find the missing medicine. At the time, of course, it is sheer panic stations. You must dread the question: "Lilly, have you got your medicine bag?" I know that sometimes we would be halfway to our destination on a day out and I would have a niggling feeling that something was not quite right. This niggling feeling would escalate to something akin to terror, as I would finally pinpoint the reason for my discomfort. No, I had not left the oven on, the door unlocked, or a window open, and yes, I had remembered spare clothes, nappies, and food for Callum, my driving license, purse, glasses, a map, and phone along with allergy free food for you, but—horror of horrors—I had forgotten to put your medicine bag in the car at the last minute. This would then result in me having to find a chemist open so I could buy some antihistamine. Your dad panics, so I dreaded confessing that we had left the bag at home as I knew that it would distress him greatly. I have tried many aids to memory through the years, from hanging the bag on the front door handle, making large signs near the door to carrying spare antihistamine in my own bag and also in the glove compartment of the car. Now that you are older and take responsibility for yourself, I panic less as I know that you are very careful about what you eat.

Since those early days, we have also discovered that you are anaphylactic to peanuts and sesame seeds. You have also had reactions to other beans (alfalfa sprouts) and some seeded fruit. You also continue to have reactions to foods that we assume are safe, although fortunately these reactions have not thus far been anaphylactic. I only know what it is like for me as a parent to deal with your allergies, and I have no idea how it must feel to you, the one dealing with the allergies. I know it has given you a fear of new foods and this is totally understandable. It has made you very careful of what you eat and an avid label reader. I am very proud of the way that you take responsibility for your allergies and are so careful to avoid foods that are dangerous to you. I encourage you, as you get older, not to get complacent about taking your medicine bag with you wherever you go. Over the years, I must have seemed like an overprotective parent to you. This is because it is a life threatening condition and I do not want anything to happen to my baby—you.

There have been some good side effects for me because of your allergies. I have to thank you for my beautifully soft hands whilst you were growing up. Before you were born, my hands were always dry and chapped during the winter months, but when you were little and I had to cream you night and day, my hands became soft and supple. Before your birth, I cooked because my family needed feeding and I rarely baked, but now of course, it is a different story. Most days, I cook food from scratch and most weeks I bake or make desserts. You have given me a new interest! I know that I enjoy my food much more now that we rarely eat processed food and I am sure that it has health benefits for the whole family. At one point, I was also making bread daily. It is only really when I have cooked or baked in this way that I can be sure that the ingredients are safe for you. It has also given me an empathy with other parents whose children have allergies and I am much more aware of the prevalence of this epidemic in our society. Of course, the downside is that supermarket trips now take me longer as I have to read every label. I have always been a bit of a slowcoach in this area, but now I really am a snail.

The biggest advantage for me came after I became a Christian, as prior to that I would sometimes become very frustrated and weary because I was awake most of the night, but was unable to actually do anything apart from rub cream on your skin. One night as I was lying on the floor by your cot, I realized that there was something I could do; I could pray. So that started my nightly encounter with God. Every situation and every problem in my life I took to God in prayer; most especially, I prayed for you and your brothers and sister and in particular, I prayed for Daniel because my heart was breaking. I know that God heard those prayers in the night watches and he continues to answer my prayers in more ways than I could ever imagine. I have had many sleepless nights since those days and I always use them to pray.

Love you,

Mum

xxxx

LETTER 3

Australia, Here We Come!

Dear Lilly,

Well, what an adventure this has been. Of course, now Australia is your home and your memories of living in the United Kingdom before we came here are probably quite dim. Arriving here was very traumatic and if I had known then what I know now, I would have done things differently, but hey, I just have to accept that I did what I did with the best of intentions. Probably because I personally was so unprepared for the move, I did not properly prepare you. Also because my life has been one of being constantly on the move, within countries, between countries, and even between continents, I thought that you would just take it all in your stride.

The move deeply unsettled you and your behavior became very erratic and unpredictable. You had screaming fits and hated going to your new school. We had picked your school on the Internet, and were so excited that you were actually going to be able to go to a Christian school. Because of our residency status at the time, we would have had to pay for you to go to the local primary school so decided that since we had to pay, we would like you to go to a Christian school. I thought that the sooner you got into school the better as it would give you some stability and routine and help you to settle into the new country quickly. So within two weeks of being here, you started your new school. Everything was different—not to mention the heat, which was overpowering. Within a few weeks of arriving here in Australia, it heated up. You were not used to the heat and started to feel faint and get headaches. It also made you very bad tempered. I, too, found the adjustment to the new school system difficult. In England, you had started to attend the local school in the village. Most of the parents personally collected their children and would all stand around in the playground or at the gates chatting waiting for the children to be dismissed. We, as parents, got to see the other children in our child's class and also meet their parents at the gate. The teachers would not let children go if their parent was not there waiting for them. It was so different in Australia. Although you were only in Year One, most of the parents used a system called "Kiss and Drop." You were all sent to a waiting area and we, the parents, queued up in cars to pick you up from the waiting area. It was very isolating for me as a parent because I did not get to meet other parents naturally. Finally I cottoned on that I could arrive early, find parking and then walk to the waiting area at the end of the day to meet you, and of course, in the morning I always parked up and took you to your classroom, but most of the other parents did not do this.

The school itself was in a semi-rural setting and therefore did not have a community feel. It was not easy to arrange for you to meet up with new friends after school because children came from far and wide to attend the school and I was soon hit with the Australian culture of *after school activities.* There was also the new language to get used to, *play-dates* had to be intricately arranged to fit in with the busy schedules of children who already had dance, music, swimming, and netball activities after school. Most of the children had been together since the beginning of kindergarten (another new word) and were also heavily committed at the weekend either to sport, family, or church activities or all three. As we did not have any other family, friends, or even a church, it took a lot of time and effort and perseverance to break into Australian culture.

You survived and made some friends, but it was not easy. From the start, you were bullied because of your eczema and had other relationship problems. There was one particular girl who was nasty to you and you told Sally during the Christmas holidays. Sally then told me and we talked about the situation. I wrote a letter to the school and I prayed a lot about the situation. I was so relieved to find that she left the school during those holidays and went elsewhere. It turned out that she had also bullied other children so, my dear, you were not the only one.

I am afraid you were stuck with mainly your dad and me, over those first couple of years here. We really struggled to fit in to Australian life and culture. We are not sporty and for obvious reasons do not drink, so did not fit into the BBQ/drinking culture here. Most weekends, we would just all pile into the car and take long drives up to the Blue Mountains with a picnic. It was the only chance your dad and I would get to have a conversation as your little brother was by this time a toddler who was very clingy to me and also had a huge sleep problem. Of course, now we know that he is autistic and that explains a lot, but then it was just totally tiring and time consuming. He had to be watched constantly as he was so unpredictable. In the car, peace reigned. He was strapped into his seat, with a couple of helicopters to play with and windows to look out of and you delighted in watching DVDs on the in-car DVD player. You put the headphones on and away we went. We also did trips to beaches and into the city. We ventured as far as Bundanoon and Canberra, but mainly, we just went up into the mountains. The Zig-zag railway became a favorite place to go.

In the first year we were here, we had visits from your dad's brother, his wife, and your paternal grandparents. Sounds fun, but mainly it wasn't as your grandma could not cope with the heat and to top it all, our air conditioner broke down during the hottest two weeks of the summer, whilst they were staying with us. My mum also came over and as she came during the cooler weather, she coped well and we had a great visit. All the time, we were struggling to make sense of why we were here and to find a church home. We visited a number of churches, some only once, some for a few weeks, some for a few months, and it took us two years to find the one we now attend. Even that has been problematic because like your first school, it is not a community church and we travel quite a distance to attend. So although we are not pioneers in the true sense of the word, every immigrant is a pioneer in a new country, crossing personal frontiers.

At the time, life seemed very hard, but I can now look back with fondness on those times that we bonded together as a family unit. We really had no one else so spent all our time with each other.

Every night after your dad finished work, he and I would take you and Callum out to a local park. You would be on your scooter, and Callum would be on his bicycle with trainer wheels.

We also started swimming together as a family and if we were not at the Blue Mountains, we were at a local leisure center, having a family swim. Good times. Do you remember them? I hope that you do and that you regard them as good times, too.

Love,

Mum

xxxx

LETTER 4

The Adolescent Years

A) ON BEING A NERD

Dear Lilly,

Today you asked me if it was okay to be a part-time nerd. You are so funny sometimes! It was 11:30 at night, on December 23, and I heard you singing in your room so came in to say goodnight. You were listening to your iPod and singing your little heart out. It made me feel all-warm inside to hear you. Then you told me that you were having trouble sleeping and asked me not to laugh if you told me what you had been doing since going to bed prior to singing. You then turned on the light and showed me a Math's revision book for two years above your current year at school, you had been sitting in bed completing some of the exercises!

"Is that a weird thing to be doing?" you asked.

I told you that at least it should prevent you from getting Alzheimer's when you were older, especially if you continued to make it a habit. It was then that you asked me if it was okay to be a part-time nerd.

My sweetheart, you want so much to be popular and beautiful and thin—above all thin—yet what you do not know is that you are indeed truly beautiful, popularity fades, and being too thin is ugly and dangerous. Of course, you are not too thin or too fat; you are just right and I want you to stay that way. I know that there is so much pressure nowadays on young girls like you to be thin and to look like models, but that is not real. We eat to live, but food is also to be savored and enjoyed. We do not need to count all our calories and measure all our food. We eat because we are hungry and need nourishment. Food is our fuel; like cars, we can't go without it. We eat good healthy food to build up our bodies and we eat a good variety of food so that we do not get bored.

Of course, I know that food has always been an issue with you because of your allergies and I am so proud of you now in the way that you approach your allergies. You are so very sensible in your attitude and always check out new foods.

Love,

Mum

xxxx

B) FACEBOOK

Dear Lilly,

Boy, girl, these letters are sure getting hard to write. I am writing them on the hoof, as they happen, raw as raw. I am writing this letter only a couple of weeks after the one I wrote after you asked me if it was okay to be a nerd. I now feel like I am writing to a completely different girl. Through all the traumas, tragedies, and triumphs I have felt and been through with your older siblings, I felt I had come to that place where I could finally communicate my true and innermost thoughts and feelings to you, my children. I actually felt that as a parent I was beginning to *do it right*. The last ten years, since I retired from teaching, I have devoted to family life.

Instead, I feel like I am facing one of the biggest challenges of my parenting skills. One day I went to bed and you were my sweet little princess, albeit sometimes an obstinate princess, but nevertheless my princess. The next morning I woke up and there was an invisible *Keep Out* sign on your bedroom door. Of course, there has been an invisible *Keep Out* sign on your door for a long time, but it never used to apply to me. It applied to an annoying little brother and children of visiting friends. It applied to a big sister looking for portable DVD players or missing chests of drawers. It has sometimes applied to your dad and I since your body started changing and you started to be more self conscious about getting dressed and undressed in front of other people. I have always felt very close to you, Lilly. You and your little brother are in reality my second family. God gave me another chance at happiness in marriage and in parenting. I have always felt very blessed to have you both as I know of many women who would love to have another child at forty and then again at forty-four.

You told me yesterday when we went for a walk that you no longer wanted to spend any time with me or anyone else in the family. I told you that it is a normal feeling as you grow older to want to spend more time with friends and less with family, but that this does not usually mean you don't want anything to do with your family. This brings me to Facebook.

Facebook is, I believe, a blessing and a curse. For me, it has been a blessing in that I have been able to keep up with your older brother and sister on another continent. It is free, quick, and accessible. I can send them a message and know that they will most likely pick it up within twenty-four hours. It has also allowed me to catch up with friends from the past that I would never otherwise see. That is the blessing side. For me, it has also been a curse in that sometimes I don't want to keep up with friends from the past. Sometimes, the past should be just that: the past.

The curse side can also be that it can become an addictive time waster and an invasion of privacy, but I really didn't see that one coming when you asked me if you could have a Facebook account.

You see the reason I did not see that coming, Lilly, is that I thought of you as being very sensible. I thought you would use Facebook in a similar way. I thought you would add a few friends, put up the occasional update, and check your friends' updates maybe once a week. In fact, I thought you would find it too time consuming, as it would take you away from your studies and piano playing. I had absolutely no idea that it would become an integral part of your life within days.

I took quite a few safeguards when I allowed you to have Facebook as a trial. I made you use an alias; I made you give me your password so I could check in on it at any time. I made you use a false picture of yourself. I made you put in a false birthdate so that it couldn't be traced to you and also that it wouldn't attract pedophiles. I made you put all your privacy settings as "friends only." I advised you that if I went on and saw anything inappropriate that you were only on trial and you could lose the privilege, albeit after warnings.

Nothing prepared me for the way you are using Facebook and your subsequent withdrawal from me since I told you that your Facebook days may be coming to an end. I had to give you several warnings over your usage. I thought that you were spending too much time on Facebook and that an addiction was developing. I have been frustrated when I have allowed you to use Facebook on my phone when we have been out, only to find that when I request my phone back you are reluctant to hand it over. I had never considered the *chat* aspect of Facebook because it is not something I use much. I am too busy to spend time on chat.

As you know, looking after your little brother is a twenty-four-hour job and I am also looking after you, your dad, and your older sister at the moment. To be honest, these summer holidays have proved quite stressful for me and I have somewhat taken my eye off the ball with you. Your sister coming back home to live at age twenty-three and then breaking her foot leaving her totally incapacitated has caused us all to have to adapt our family living. Having another person dependent on me has meant that there has been less time to go around for the rest of you. In addition, all your food needs are so different that buying, preparing, and serving food has become a major issue in our house. So in a way, I was happy that you seemed to be amusing yourself and was not really aware that you were spending so much time on Facebook. This holiday season has been disappointing for me. I had been hoping that your older brother would be able to spend Christmas with us and also that one of your uncles and aunties would come for a visit from the United Kingdom. I was so busy before Christmas that all my usual planning, charts, menus, etc. just haven't been done. Just when I thought that you were okay, having settled into your new school and made some friends, I am now wondering just what exactly is going on with you.

You always look so sad. I think you are being bullied on Facebook, but are not really aware that this is happening. This is because I have seen some of the messages people have sent you and your responses to them. I think that you are chatting with people inappropriately and are going on late at night when I think you have gone upstairs to bed.

When I told you that I was thinking of making you close your Facebook account, you had such a severe reaction that it really worried me. You said you were really angry, told me to get out of your room, and then went downstairs and started banging around the kitchen. I had never really seen you like that before. I found it quite scary. Of course, we have had our moments; you have never liked not getting your own way, but who does?

We have now agreed that you and I will sit down and go through your Facebook account and I will write a contract of use that you will sign if you wish to continue to use the account. To be honest, I have only checked your account a couple of times and as I was thinking of going through it again, I checked it again today. What I have seen has made me reconsider and unless I get the response I am looking for from you, I think it is going to have to be suspended now until we get time to sit down and go through the account. Facebook is a public arena and we have to be very careful what we put on it.

I can see that the teenage years are not going to be easy for us. I feel I have put in the right foundations this time, but time will tell. I have always been open with you. I have tried to teach you about life. I have tried to teach you and not let any subject be taboo. I have tried to answer your questions about God, about friendships, about puberty, about relationships; in short, I have tried to be more open than my parents were with me. I have tried to be there for you and to be your advocate at school and in general. I know that it has been hard for you coming to terms with your allergies where every food is a potential danger. I know that you have found moving very traumatic and we have moved a lot.

Just know that I love you and that I only want the best for you. I love the fact that we are doing devotions again together at night and I hope that this will continue. I am finding it a little scary to see what you have written on Facebook as I didn't know what you were thinking or that you were even thinking about the things you write about. It is such a hard time of transition from child to adult; from dependency to independence; from feeling that your parents know everything to finding out that they don't. You are going through a metamorphosis, not in a literal way, but in an emotional way. You are realizing that there is a great big world out there and you want to be part of it, but we, as parents, are trying to protect you from the big world out there and wanting you to be safe and secure. We know that all too soon, you will have to fend for yourself and make your own decisions and we know that whilst it gives freedom, with freedom come responsibility and consequences.

So sorry, Lilly, that I let you try Facebook too early, and sorry, Lilly, but it looks like I will have to withdraw that privilege from you for a while.

Love,

Mum

xxxx

P.S. Well, I did withdraw you from Facebook for a while and since then you have temporarily closed down your own account voluntarily. I think it is good to do this from time to time and have a rest from too much social networking. I still think that you spend too much time on Facebook, but more and more, I am realizing that it is not just an issue with you, but with our society in general. We spend less time face-to-face with our friends and more time on Facebook!

At your age, your older brothers and sister were meeting up with their friends on street corners and hanging out. Your generation chooses to *hang out* on Facebook and on Skype. At least it is free! Plus, I know where you are and can see what you are doing. I believe that mostly you are sensible about your use. You talk to people you know and stay on too long, but what is the point in being a teenager if you don't spend too long talking to your friends? A little more wisdom is still needed in your use, but I believe that will come with time. The only thing I would suggest is you shorten your friends list and get rid of famous people or sites that are just trying to sell you something or get you to be their fan and just keep it to personal friends. Always remember that what you write or post on Facebook is in the public domain; nothing is private, so do not write anything that would prejudice your teachers, other friends, or future employers against you. Protect yourself from Cyber bullying by instantly removing people from your friends list if they send you nasty messages. Also don't be a cyber bully yourself—don't send nasty messages to others, no matter how much they have annoyed or upset you. Don't invade their personal, private, safe place—home—and don't allow them to invade yours.

I think it is so typical of you that you have placed a piece of card over your webcam and keep it stuck there so that people cannot remotely access your computer and watch you when you least suspect it. Wish I had thought of that one first!

C) FRIENDS

Dear Lilly,

Hot topic: we all want them, we all need them, but it is really hard choosing them. Throughout your young life, you have struggled in this area. You seem to find it really easy to make friends, but keeping them seems to elude you. I remember telling you a few years ago that in order to have friends, you should be a friend and this still holds. Friendships are all about give and take, listening and sharing, and putting other people first. It is a natural thing that some friendships taper off, for example if you move away from an area or a school. If you stop coming into contact with certain friends often that friendship will fade.

I guess, as we get older, new friendships are based on common interests. Your world is a different world from the world I grew up in. Even taking into account the normal generational gap, because I had an unusual childhood myself, was institutionalized from the age of four and had little so-called normal family life, we can't really compare our upbringings or life experiences. In my experience, there are very few friends that are lifelong friends. This is not just because I have moved about so much; it is also because some friendships are for certain times in our lives. It is not that they are not real friends—they are just friends for a season. For example, when I was a teacher, I had lots of other friends who were teachers. I socialized with the people I worked with. We had our work in common. When I was a member of a trade union and political party in the United Kingdom, I had friends who were also members of that trade union and political party. We had common goals and ideals. Now that I have a son who is autistic, I have friends who are also parents of an autistic child. We share the common experience that is parenting a child who is autistic. We listen and can relate to what the other parents are going through and they in turn listen to us and we know they can hear what we are saying.

I know that you think that ever since Callum's diagnosis, I see autism in everyone and I guess, in a way, all of us have a few of the traits to some degree or another. Your dad relates to the diagnosis and believes that he, too, is on the Autism Spectrum. It certainly explains a lot about the way he is. You know, too, that I think that you have a mild version of Asperger's Syndrome, but I am acutely aware that you strongly disagree. I wish you could embrace it and work with it. There are many people who are happy Aspies, who recognize and celebrate their difference and having done that, it gives them a whole new perspective on life. The diagnosis would certainly explain a lot of your behaviors, especially the trauma you went through when we moved to Australia. It also explains your perfectionist streak and your ability to excel and persevere with tasks you enjoy. It turns stubbornness into single-mindedness. Enough of that. This is something we have talked about at length and I guess we just have to agree to disagree. You have confessed to me that you have a lot of obsessions and feel that you suffer from OCD and you have also told me that for the majority of the time, you feel very depressed and angry and think you are different from other people. You have very low self-esteem and it seems nothing I can say to the contrary changes your opinion of yourself. You are a lovely young lady with many good qualities.

On another topic, ideally the person you marry will be a lifelong friend and I have to say that your dad, my husband, is my best friend. I love him and he loves me despite the fact that we are not blind to each other's faults. I know you say that you never want to get married and that you never want to have children, but you may change your mind when you get older.

In addition, I have certain friends from my childhood that I still consider my friends although I hardly ever see them. When we do see each other, it is as though the time since we last saw each other has melted away and the friendship is still there. These would be other missionary kids like my friend in Christchurch and friends now in Canada and the United States. These friendships were formed in the adversity of being together in boarding school that was run by a headmaster with sadistic tendencies and separated from our parents at a young age, of being brought up in a culture alien to our parents' culture and then having to reintegrate into our parents' culture. We know without having to explain to each other what our schooldays were like. We share the common bond of having to forge a life for ourselves without the backing of close family in a new and alien culture, which is assumed to be our culture.

Outside of these friendships, all my friends are other Christians and we are friends because we share a common faith. In fact, I regard my Christian friends as more than friends; they are my brothers and sisters. As you get older and have a family, you also realize that your family comes before your friends, but at your age, often having friends seems more important than being loved and cherished by your family. There is so much time to be grown up and responsible for your own life; enjoy this time when you have parents to provide for you and guide you.

There are other differences, too. The explosion of social networking has changed the way friendships are formed and maintained, in irrevocable ways. In the past, you maintained friendships by meeting up with your friends and doing stuff together. Nowadays, friendships are also maintained through mobile phones and social media, such as Facebook. Now that you are back on Facebook, you need to watch out for its pitfalls. I thought it was so sensible a couple of months ago when you voluntarily came off for a few weeks because in the same way that it can increase contact with your friends, it can also increase feelings of isolation and rejection as you get to see what all your *friends* are doing with each other and you weren't invited!

Having true friends is not the same as being in the popular group in school. Real friends like you for who you are, not whom you are friends with or what you look like. With real friends, you can be yourself; you don't have to hide who you really are and you don't have to pretend.

I encourage you to keep working at your friendships, to believe that you are a nice person, who is worth knowing, and treat other people the way you would like to be treated. It is hard, but don't worry about how many friends you have. Above all, don't be persuaded to do things you know are wrong or you are not comfortable with, in order to gain popularity. It is not worth it. Pursue the things that give you pleasure, such as your music, and as you pursue these things and develop your talents, you will find others that are on the same path as you. Quiet confidence is the key. Also start talking and keep talking. Share with me what is going on in your life. I am here for you. Sorry if all I ever seem to do is tell you to tidy your room, do your homework, practice the piano, finish up on the computer, cut your telephone call short, walk the dog, sort out your clothes, wash the dishes, and hurry up and get ready. Mothering is more than this and I know that I am often guilty of the above. I am trying to learn from past mistakes and see through your masquerade to the lovely girl that is you. I am trying to hang in there even when you scream that you hate me and that I never let you do anything you want. I know inside that there is a hurting girl and that I am not really the reason for the hurt; I am just there receiving the effects. I also know that inside there is a girl who wants to be grown up and make her own decisions, but who isn't quite there yet.

I am looking forward to seeing you achieve your potential in life and become the beautiful woman that I know you will be, inside and out. Most of all, I want to see you allowing God's grace to work in your life and letting your head knowledge of Jesus become your heart knowledge. I want to see you loving the Lord your God with all your heart and with all your soul and with all your might and I want to see you serving only him, but that, sweetheart, is your choice.

Love,

Mum

xxxx

LETTERS TO CALLUM

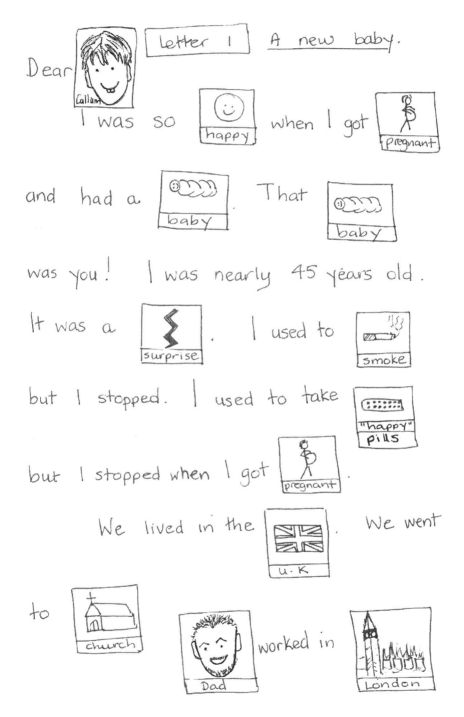

Dear [Callum]

Letter 1 · A new baby.

I was so [happy] when I got [pregnant] and had a [baby]. That [baby] was you! I was nearly 45 years old. It was a [surprise]. I used to [smoke] but I stopped. I used to take ["happy" pills] but I stopped when I got [pregnant]. We lived in the [U.K]. We went to [church]. [Dad] worked in [London].

but we lived in the . He

was away during the week and home

at the weekend. 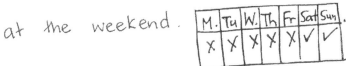.

You had 2 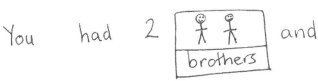 and

2 already. was 17

and lived in Scotland with his mum.

 was also 17 and lived nearby

with his friend's family. I was sad

that he did not live with us.

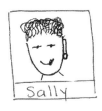 and 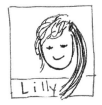 lived with us.

You were a very baby. I

stayed at home with you whilst

 and 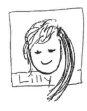 went to school.

 was in the 1st year of school

and 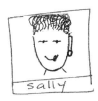 was in the last year of

school.

When you were 10 months old we went on an aeroplane to visit my sister in Canada. It was a lot of fun

I was very happy to have my 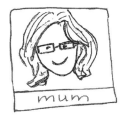 baby

with me 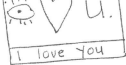 I love you

mum

XOXO XOXO.

Goodbye 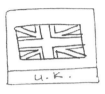 Hello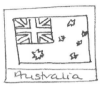

Dear 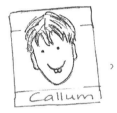 ,

When you were 2 years old,

 got a job in 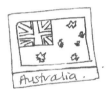 We

decided to move because he would

be paid and he would live at

home 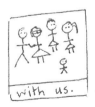 . and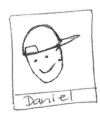

did not come with us. (☹   I was sad.)

It was a very long journey. We left

in Wales on Friday morning

and arrived in Sydney, Australia on

Sunday night.   I was very tired.

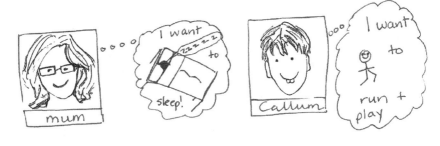

You did not want to sleep!

Being in a new country was a bit

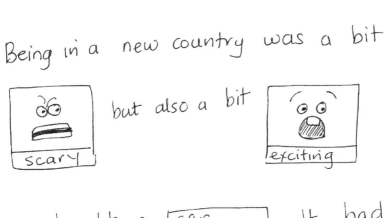 but also a bit

We bought a 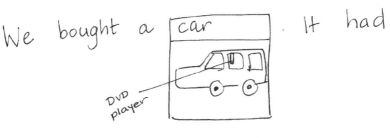. It had

8 seats and a DVD player.

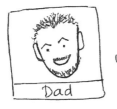 went to work with

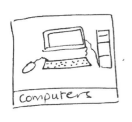 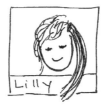 went to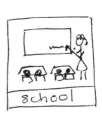

and 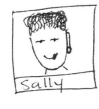 got a job making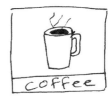

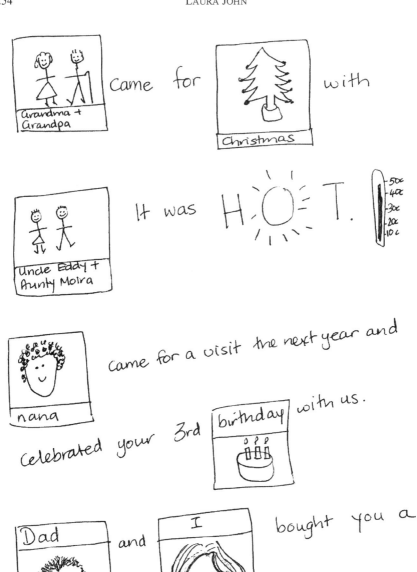

Grandma + Grandpa Came for Christmas with

Uncle Eddy + Aunty Moira It was HOT.

nana Came for a visit the next year and Celebrated your 3rd birthday with us.

Dad and I bought you a

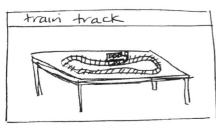 but you did not play

with it. Instead you played with the

 that was a gift from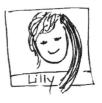

You loved the helicopter and would not
let it go. It was the 1st of many
planes and helicopters.

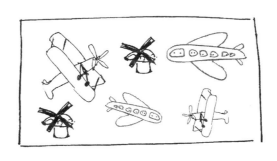

From then on you lived and breathed aeroplanes and helicopters.

We lived under a flight path and whenever you heard a plane, you would look for it in the sky.

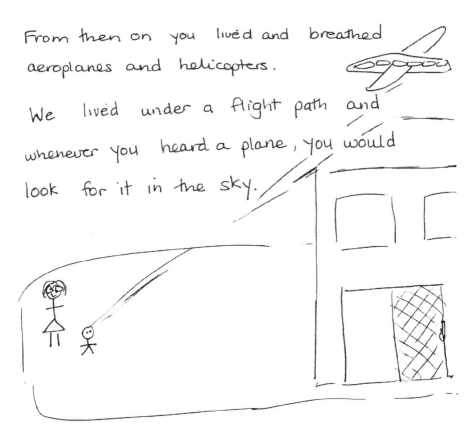

You also loved to watch DVD's about fighter planes over and over again

In 2007 we became permanent residents of 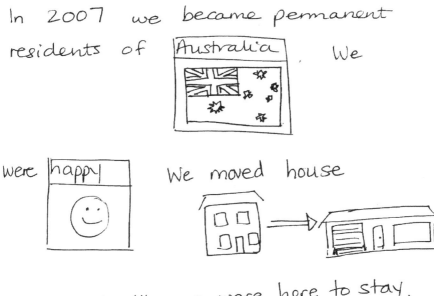. We

were 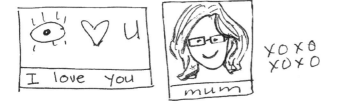 We moved house

It lööked like we were here to stay.

I love you

mum

XOXO
XOXO

Letter 3

An a 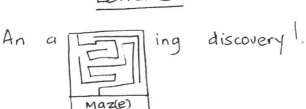 ing discovery !.

Maz(e)

Dear 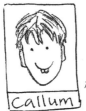 Everyone is different and

Callum ,

special. 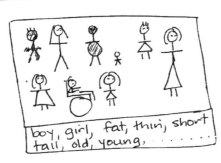 One day

boy, girl, fat, thin, short
tall, old, young, ...

we found out that you 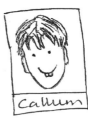 were

Callum

very, very special.

You started going to "Prep" 2 days a week at the same 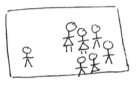 as

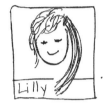 You did not play with the other children very much.

You wanted to go on the computer.

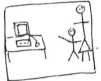 You did not look at the teacher 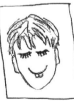 and did not say

"Hi". You were very shy. The teacher was 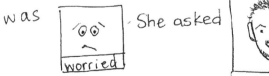 She asked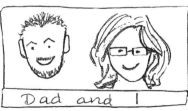

lots of questions . I took you to see

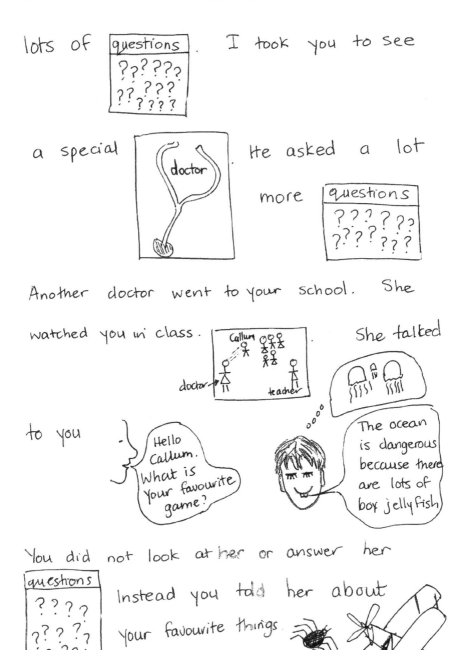

a special doctor . He asked a lot

more questions

Another doctor went to your school. She

watched you in class. . She talked

to you

Hello Callum. What is your favourite game?

The ocean is dangerous because there are lots of box jellyfish

You did not look at her or answer her questions Instead you told her about your favourite things.

Everyone decided that you were a very special person. They gave it a name they said

is AUTISTIC.

Callum

Now had lots of questions

Dad and I

We found out you have a very clever brain

You think in pictures

your sense of smell is very strong

your sense of taste is very strong

It works differently from most other people.

There is so much stuff squashed into your brain that you find it hard to remember things. or to sort out what to say.

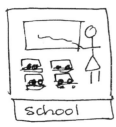 is very hard for you. So many sights, sounds, smells and people. So much time doing things you

hate. like 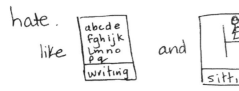 and 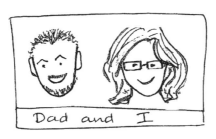 are very

proud of you. We know you will succeed in what you want to do as you have a lot of something called. PERSEVERANCE.

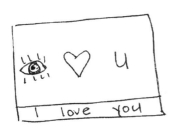 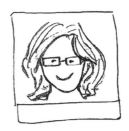

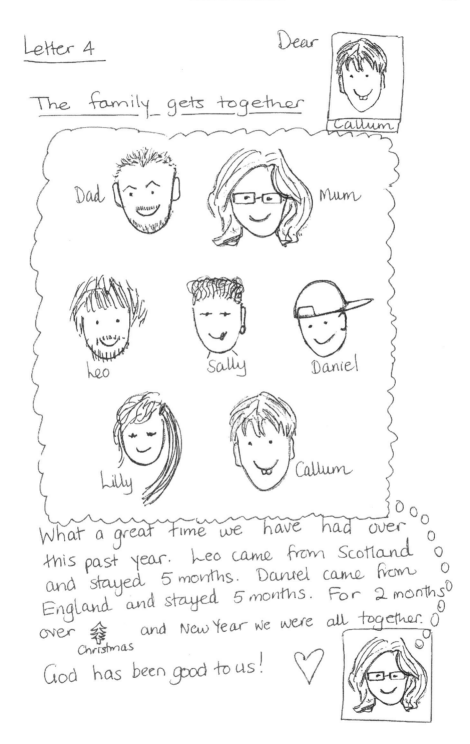

Letter 4

Dear

Callum

The family gets together

Dad

Mum

Leo

Sally

Daniel

Lilly

Callum

What a great time we have had over this past year. Leo came from Scotland and stayed 5 months. Daniel came from England and stayed 5 months. For 2 months over 🎄 Christmas and New Year we were all together.

God has been good to us!

5

Renewal of Vows

Remembering Our First Wedding

Dear Leo, Daniel, Sally, Lilly, and Callum,

I can't believe that we will finally all be together again, in the same place. This has been my dream for the last five years. This is what I have prayed for, longed for, and sought after. As a birth mother, I have wanted for us all to be together in harmony for so long, and as a step-mother, I have wanted you, Leo, to be part of this because your dad is my soul mate, my other half, and without you the picture would not be complete.

As you know Leroy/dad and I have been planning to renew our wedding vows for some time now. When we first got married, we had no real belief in God and we were basically just living for the moment. For this reason, we chose to get married in a registry office and actually looking back, we did not give the ceremony or the marriage much thought; we just did it. We obviously thought that marriage was the way forward for our relationship and did not just want to live together, so I guess that was a start in the right direction.

Leo, Daniel, and Sally, you will probably remember our wedding differently from me and from each other. I find that when I look back on events of my childhood, I often view the same event very differently from my sister and parents. This is because the bare facts are the same for everyone, but the way the event impacts us differs. I was in love and so minimized everything that went wrong. I was not really aware of any of the dramas faced by any of the guests. I was not really aware of the impact that our wedding and marriage was having on our children.

265

I remember talking to you, Daniel and Sally, about getting married and asking if you were happy about it. At the time, you both said that you were happy that I was getting married and both seemed to like and get on with Leroy. We had moved to a first-floor apartment in South East London. I had been in the process of buying the property when Leroy and I met and he moved in a couple of months after we met. Leroy was also in the process of buying a new flat in Surrey when we met and it was not finished, so he moved in with us whilst waiting for completion by the builders. It was during this time that we decided to get married. You both seemed to get on with Leroy pretty well and there did not seem to be any dramas. At the time, you were spending every other weekend with your dad or your dad's family and the rest of the time, life seemed to be continuing as before. Leroy was working on the other side of London and was not involved in the day-to-day parenting of you both—that was still completely up to me. Looking back, he was more of a treat supplier at that time. On the weekends that you were with us, he arranged outings to theme parks or days out at the beach or swimming. If he was going to buy beer at the off-license, he always took one or both of you along and treated you to sweets or a soft drink. He bought a couple of second hand TVs so that you could each have a TV.

Strangely enough, a couple of events really impacted on my decision to commit to marriage at that time. The first was that Princess Diana died in an horrific car crash in Paris; the second was that Leroy, Sally, and I were involved in a horrific car crash ourselves whilst I was driving.

As usual, death makes us reassess life. Of course, I did not know Princess Diana so felt no personal grief—rather shock that her fame and wealth had made no difference. The media, however, is such that it makes us feel as if we know famous people, so when they die it does not seem as if a stranger has died. We connect and in a way feel loss although we, in fact, have not lost anything. Particularly with Princess Diana, we, the public, were made to feel as though we were sharing in her life as her every move was recorded by the press. We knew which gym she went to, where she shopped and spent her holidays, how she felt about her marriage and its eventual breakdown. We watched her bringing up her two sons and were spies on her relationships. We knew her passions and her problems, her likes and dislikes. In my case, her death made me think about my own life. My reasoning was, I could die any day, any time (my own car accident reinforced the fragility of life and completely traumatized me, and I truly felt as though I had seen the jaws of death) so why wait to get married? I was in love. It was my own father's death that had prompted my move to London in order that you two could be nearer to your own father. I also wanted to share my life with someone and felt that that someone was Leroy.

Death is no respecter of persons. Apart from suicide, no one really controls their death; it is always ever just around the corner for all of us. None of us are invincible or immune. Life was a different matter and I felt I needed to be pro-active rather than reactive. Make a decision, make a change, commit, and get married. Leroy and I both shared the same views about marriage. Neither of us was really in favor of living together, so before we really had time to think, we were down at the council offices booking a date for the wedding. Neither of us had any money saved up. Teacher's wages are not high and the cost of living in London is extortionate. This along with the fact that I had two mortgages and my car had been written off as a result of the accident meant I not only had no savings, but also was in debt. So we booked a wedding, but had no money to splash out on a reception or a honeymoon.

The ceremony itself was pretty nondescript and in many ways a bit of a farce. The taxis we had ordered did not turn up, so we all got to the venue (Council offices in Bromley, Kent) in dribs and drabs and some close family arrived at the end of the ceremony. Daniel, you laughed uncontrollably throughout the short ceremony as my sister had unwittingly allowed you to have a cola, which made you hyper.

Leo, I had never met your grandma before the actual wedding day and she and your dad had not spoken to each other for two years prior to that date. I did not feel that I was being welcomed into the family at all, as only one of your dad's five brothers came to the wedding and at the end of the short ceremony, your grandma's words to me were as follows: "I wish you luck. You must be old enough to know what you are doing."

Not exactly the warmest welcome, you will admit.

At the time, I laughed it off and was just glad that she was there as I thought it was important to have parents at a wedding. Looking back, our families must have been wary. I would not be surprised if some of our family and friends thought that we were being very unwise. We first met in June and by November of the same year, we were getting married. I am sure a lot was said behind the scenes about how foolish we were and I suspect that most people at the wedding only gave our marriage a few years before it folded. I know that my cousin Carol, who is also my closest friend, took Leroy aside at the reception and warned him not to mistreat me in any way. She was worried because he didn't have a job when we actually got married and she was concerned that I would end up supporting him financially, as I had my first husband. She needn't have worried on that score as Leroy has supported me financially all the time we have been married.

So that was our first wedding. Leroy now tells me that he was drunk at the time (I did not realize). We stayed one night in a bed and breakfast and then commenced our married life together without really knowing each other at all. There were, however, a couple of things that we discussed: loyalty and children.

As both of us had been cheated on in our marriages and were both deeply hurt by the unfaithfulness of our previous spouses, we put loyalty to each other as our number one requirement. In fact, you could say that it was our only priority. I had decided that I would never argue about washing up or other household chores. The most important thing to me was that Leroy was faithful to me in word and deed, that he would not go off with other women, and that he would love only me. He said that it was the same for him.

As for children, Leroy passionately wanted more children; I was not convinced. I remember saying that if we had more children and ever split up, he had to know that he would be looking after them. Having just spent six years as a single parent, I did not want to repeat this process. Anyone who has ever been a single parent will know how daunting a task it is. At the time, my career was just taking off and I was gaining in confidence as a teacher, although I loved my children I was not actually sure that I could cope with more. I knew the twenty-four/seven commitment it required and I rather selfishly wanted to pursue my career. Of course, I was also struggling financially and could not see how I could continue to work and have children, but I knew I needed to work to eat. So there was a bit of a difference in our expectations. I was aware that Leroy desperately wanted more children and he was aware that he would have to persuade me, as I was not keen. In the end, we just decided to get married and worry about whether or not we would have children afterwards. I guess Leroy decided that he wanted to marry me more than he wanted more children and I decided that I wanted to marry him enough to consider having more children after we married. The rest is history and I am so glad that we did have more children, as I love you all dearly. In fact, I think that the fact that we have children together is the thing that has kept us together in difficult times. We both believe that children need both their parents and are committed to not repeating the mistakes we made with the older ones.

So there you have it; we talked about loyalty and children and when I look back on our marriage thus far, that is what it has all been about. Leroy has been the most loyal husband I could ever wish to have and you two youngest children have been the fruit of our union.

As for the wedding itself, I have never been one to make a fuss and mostly don't like being the center of attention. I bought a purple dress off the rack for forty pounds and on the day, my sister bought me a lacy black jacket. Leroy had a new red shirt, which he wore with his Marilyn Monroe tie (it matched her lips) and his leather waistcoat with tassels. We had no flowers, special music, hairdos, or makeup. We had no special vows that we wrote for each other and no reception afterwards—just a meal in a local pub and everyone had to pay for their own food.

So that was our first wedding.

Love,

Mum/Laura

xxxx

LETTER TWO

Commitment at the Beach

Dear Leo, Daniel, Sally, Lilly, and Callum,

You will know by reading the other letters I have written to each of you that our marriage has had its ups and downs already and no doubt more will come, but renewing our vows was very, very special to us, even more special because you shared in the day.

Firstly, I need to say the biggest thank you of my life to all of you for making the day so special. The most amazing thing about the day for me was the way you all wanted to please Leroy and me by making it the kind of day we wanted. You wore the clothes we had chosen for you and in every way, you all sought to please. You stood where we wanted you to stand; you all took part in the ceremony and backed us up. All of you seemed genuinely excited about what we were doing and were very supportive. You all looked stunning: Leo in his kilt, matching Leroy in his, Sally and Lilly in your matching Zara floral prints, and Daniel and Callum in your traditional white shirts with black ties. I loved the verses that all you boys read and Callum, I was particularly proud of you for overcoming your shyness to read your verses in front of all the guests. I loved the poems that you girls read. Sally, I am honored that you chose to read your favorite poem at the renewal and Lilly, I loved the poem that you composed.

To me, it was as much about Leroy and I making our vows of love before God as it was standing there with all of our children in one place, at one time, and united in love showing the world and whoever cared to look on, that we were a family and that we loved each other. When I think of all our family has been through thus far, it is truly a miracle that we were all together in such a situation. I can't really say enough; it was a dream-come-true for me. I will never, never forget that day. Whatever happens in the future, that day will be etched in my memory as the best. For that day, all the heartache faded, all the past receded, all the pain was dimmed. You guys made me feel really special; whatever I asked you to do, you did.

Our lives are not perfect and each of us is facing difficult situations, times of decision, and times of trial, but on that day it did not matter to me. I was truly able to live for the day—oh, and not forgetting the night—it was so amazing of you all to free up Leroy and me to spend the night together in a hotel. You were so generous in giving of your time to look after each other. We thought we were going to have to rush back in the morning, but no, you told us to take our time and not rush back. You will never know how much I appreciated the willing offer of your time on that day. It was one of the most relaxing mornings of my life, knowing that Callum was in good hands and that you were all willing to be part of his day so that Leroy and I could have our day.

There is much else I could say about the day and I certainly have other people to thank, but the fact that my cousin Carol was also able to be there and be a part of our day was so special to me, especially because no one else from our extended families could be there.

In the middle of three weeks of cloudy skies, rain, and thunderstorms, there opened up a beautiful afternoon of sunshine, warmth, and blue skies and it was the afternoon of our celebrations. God is so good. I truly feel that he is interested even in the small details of our lives and I feel that as he is in charge of the weather, he totally blessed us that afternoon with glorious sunshine. It was the icing on the cake. I was worried that there would be a thunderstorm as the vows were outside, but Leroy remained confident that God would bless us with good weather. That is one of the things I love about Leroy, his ability to be sure of a good outcome in certain situations.

Of course, I was also overcome that Leroy chose to read Proverbs 31 to me and that he told me that he thought I was like the wife it describes. That was such an honor; sometimes in the humdrum of life we women can feel so much that the work that we do around the house and with the children goes unnoticed and is not appreciated. We all know that it is often only when it is not done that it is noticed. I did not know what he was going to say or read as we had decided this would be a secret, to make the day have a little bit of the unknown in it. So it was a surprise when he read those verses. It was so wonderful to hear him tell me that he loved me in front of all of you and in front of all our guests and any other beachgoers who were watching and listening on the day. It is easy to say all these things at the start of a relationship, but it is something else to still be able to say them a few years down the line, especially after some of the things that we have been through as a couple and as a family.

On that day God exchanged for me:

Beauty for Ashes

The Oil of Joy for Mourning and

The Garment of Praise for the Spirit of Heaviness

—Isaiah 61:3 (NKJ version)

Epilogue

Dear readers,

I hope that this book has both enlightened and encouraged you. Since these letters were written, things have moved on for my family. Leo is back in Scotland, living with his grandma, working hard and saving up with a view to returning to Australia on a more permanent basis. Daniel is back in England, attending an Urban Evangelism course, pursuing his music and he, too, plans to return to Australia, sooner rather than later, to live and work. Sally has moved out of home and she is avidly pursuing her career. Lilly is still at school and remains in the throes of teenage angst, but is pursuing her piano and guitar playing and is in her school band. Callum never ceases to amaze us and his current obsession is a computer game called Minecraft. Leroy has given up IT and is now a pastor at the church that we have attended for six years. He is also fervently continuing his theological studies. On a more serious note, he is now battling a serious heart condition and has had to undergo major open-heart surgery, but that is another story. As for me, I am, of course, by God's grace, continuing to write and attempting to be the mother and wife that God wants me to be.

—Laura John

Printed in Australia
AUOC01n1534070813
257313AU00001B/1/P

9 781625 164087